TEST  YOUR DIET SENSE

TRUE OR FALSE?

1. Calories don't count.
2. A crash diet is an excellent way to begin a weight loss program.
3. Exercise is unimportant in weight control.
4. Eating more in the morning will put on less weight than eating food in the evening.
5. Hot foods, such as soups, will leave you with a greater feeling of satisfaction because they take longer to swallow and absorb.
6. Boiling, broiling, baking and steaming are the best techniques for preparing food.
7. Toasting bread reduces its calorie count.
8. Since protein is the most important nutritional requirement of the body, high protein diets are the healthiest.
9. Margarine is 100% fat.
10. Certain foods, such as grapefruit, can burn up calories.

Answers: 1. false; **2.** false; **3.** false; **4.** false; **5.** true; **6.** true; **7.** false; **8.** false; **9.** true; **10.** false.

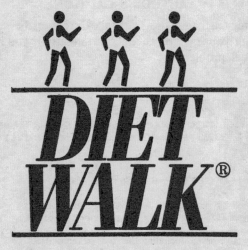

DIET WALK®

The Doctor's F*A*S*T* 3-Day Superdiet

Fred A. Stutman, M.D.

PUBLISHED BY POCKET BOOKS NEW YORK

AUTHOR'S CAUTION

Before you begin the Dietwalk® program be sure to consult your own physician, particularly if you have a medical problem.

POCKET BOOKS, a division of Simon & Schuster, Inc.
1230 Avenue of the Americas, New York, N.Y. 10020

Copyright © 1983 by Fred A. Stutman, M.D.

Published by arrangement with Medical Manor Books®
Library of Congress Catalog Card Number: 83-61033

ISBN: 0-671-61450-9

First Pocket Books printing April 1987

10 9 8 7 6 5 4 3 2 1

MEDICAL MANOR BOOKS® is the registered
trademark of Manor House Publications, Inc.

DIETWALK® is the registered trademark
of Fred A. Stutman, M.D.

POCKET and colophon are registered trademarks
of Simon & Schuster, Inc.

Cover design by Amy King

Printed in the U.S.A.

To
Suzanne
Robert, Rhonda, Craig
Irene and George

ACKNOWLEDGMENTS

EDITOR:
Dr. Suzanne T. Stutman

MANUSCRIPT PREPARATION:
Patricia McGarvey

WORD PROCESSING:
Hadassah Freifelder: The Automated Typist, Phila., PA

OFFICE STAFF:
Sheryl Bartkus, Ann Birchler, Maryanne Johnston, Linda Wilson

MEDICAL CHARTS & ILLUSTRATIONS:
Carnation Healthcare Services; Family Practice News; Kellogg Co.; McGraw-Hill Publishers; Medical Times, a Romaine Pierson Publication; Medical Tribune; Oxford University Press; The Physician and Sportsmedicine, a McGraw-Hill Publication; U.S.V. Laboratories, Inc.

PRODUCT PERMISSION:
Egg Beaters®, Fleischmann Division, Nabisco Brands, Inc.; Fibermed®, The Purdue Frederick Co.; Kellogg® Products, a division of Kellogg Co. Inc.; Pam®, Boyle-Midway Division, American Home Products Inc.; Superpretzel®, J & J Snack Foods, Inc.

PUBLISHER:
Medical Manor Books, Philadelphia, PA

*Hippocrates,
the founder of medicine,
stated over 2,000 years ago that
"Regular exercise is man's best friend."*

Contents

Introduction

There have been literally thousands of diet books and hundreds of fitness books written over the past decade. Many of these were written by non-professionals whose information was based on inaccurate, and, in many cases, erroneous medical and physiological facts.

The **diet business** is just that, a big business in the U.S. which preys on the millions of Americans who are waiting for the ultimate solution to their weight problems. Diet promoters constantly release new diet gimmicks and fad diets which often are based on non-scientific facts, and which contain just enough information to make them sound plausible. With very little exception, most of these diet gimmicks and quick weight loss programs all have one thing in common— they are potentially hazardous to your health if continued for any prolonged period of time.

The **fitness boom** has a more recent origin in the U.S., dating back to the early 1970's. During this period, the jogging craze hit America, and people by the thousands succumbed to this frantic sport with its inherent injuries and disabilities. There is no getting away from the basic medical fact that jogging is potentially hazardous to your health. Injuries, accidents, disabilities, and on rare occasion, even deaths, have been reported as a result of this strenuous exercise.

13

In the past five years we have seen an entire industry develop comprised of weight-loss centers, health spas, fitness clubs and diet clinics. All of these programs promise instant weight loss and fitness results, provided that you are able to keep up with the payments and don't die of exhaustion, starvation or boredom.

DIETWALK®: THE DR.'S F*A*S*T* 3-DAY WEIGHT-LOSS & FITNESS PLAN was originally written for my patients who, like you, were tired of expensive, time-consuming diet plans and fitness programs. All too often these gimmick diet plans end in frustration with additional rebound weight gain. And how many of you have the time or energy to devote to back-breaking, foot-pounding, exhausting exercises in order to achieve the "mythical physical fitness award"? This program is the first lifetime system for weight control and physical fitness without strenuous exercises or fad diet plans.

THE DR.'S F*A*S*T* 3-DAY DIETWALK® is a unique concept in the annals of dieting. There are no calories or grams to count, no foods to weigh or measure, no special foods to buy or prepare, and no starvation tactics to endure. This inexpensive diet program will enable you to stay thin and trim for a lifetime with a minimum of effort on your part. In addition to keeping you thin, the diet provides a built-in protective mechanism against many diseases and degenerative conditions of aging that affect us all. Here at last is a safe effective diet, that's as good for your insides as it is for your figure. This program is designed to help you lose weight, stay thin, keep fit and live longer.

This is the F*IRST A*MERICAN S*UPER DIET* & *fitness plan ever developed and the last one you will ever need!*

1

HOW TO LOSE WEIGHT WITHOUT DIETING

THE ENDLESS DIET

How many times have you started on that endless Monday morning diet, swearing to yourself that this time would be for keeps? How many new diet fads or crazes have you marched to the tune of, until, out of desperation, you are forced to once more join the legion of the overweight? It seems that no matter how good you try to be, how carefully you try to follow your diet, losing the pounds and keeping them off becomes a never-ending battle.

Diet books are being released and consumed almost as fast as we consume our food. The end result is always the same. The books provide an endless array of gimmicks, gadgets, secret tips, and pointers for "rapid weight loss." Most are generally **nutritionally unsound** and in many cases are detrimental to our health and well-being. However, no matter what non-medical or pseudo-physiological basis these diet books are based on, they always occupy one or two places on the best-seller list. The reason: most of us are seeking the ultimate, easy, non-fattening, rapid weight-loss program. Well, face facts; such a program **doesn't exist!** This kind of diet always ends in a fizzle of boring, monotonous food preparation and food avoidance. Can I eat this food? Can I have that on my diet? How many calories does it have? How many grams are in that cracker?

Well, you get the point. Your life becomes obsessed with foods, calories, fats, proteins, carbohydrates, etc. These diets take all forms, but in general, most of them deal in half-truths. They give enough basic nutritional and physiological information to make them appear sound, but if you examine them carefully, you will find that they all have the same basic facts: you can't stay on them for the rest of your life, because they are physiologically and biochemically unsound. The body chemistry can be fooled initially, but after a short period of time, our bodies begin to react or rebel against the nonsense that these diets proclaim. The majority of these diets ignore the nutritional requirements and the health of the dieter.

NON-DIET DISCOVERY

Anthropologists have unearthed by their studies a near-perfect non-diet discovery for weight loss and maintenance. *Pre-historic man* was by all intents and purposes first a tree dweller and later a land-rover and hunter. By reconstructing prehistoric bones, it became possible to reconstruct the physical build of these men. Lo and behold, what we have is the picture of a lean, trim individual. He walked, ran and climbed everywhere, unless he was sleeping. Although he ate whenever he could, he stayed thin because he burned up whatever food he ate. In other words, his *activity level* was equal to or greater than his *intake of food*. Prehistoric man was the first man to demonstrate the fact that **walking** was the ideal weight control and fitness program.

What are we to conclude from these unusual findings? Well, first and foremost, it is the amount of *walking* that we do that controls and maintains our *weight* and *body build*. If we walk too little we will gain weight, and if we walk more we will lose weight. It almost sounds too easy to be true. Here is a weight reduction plan without actually dieting and a fitness program without strenuous exercises. Now, for the first time in your life, you can lose or maintain weight comfortably and still enjoy your favorite foods without rigid diets or starvation tactics.

WEIGHT LOSS WITHOUT DIETING?

How would you like to be able to lose weight without dieting, or be able to maintain your desired weight without any dietary restrictions? Sounds impossible, doesn't it! Well, believe it or not, medical science has rediscovered a way to accomplish these facts without the use of nuclear physics, computer science, biochemical or genetic engineering; neither does it involve complicated, hazardous weight reduction gimmicks or fad diets. The answer is a basic fact in human physiology: **WALKING!**

Weight loss without dieting? Impossible, you say! The truth of the matter is that it is not only possible but it is very practical. In fact, it is the only method by which you can lose and maintain your weight for the rest of your life. How would you like to eat whatever you want and indulge yourself on occasion if you so desire? Well, **THE WEIGHT-LOSS WALKING PROGRAM** will enable you finally to embark upon the only permanent **NON-DIET** anywhere in the world.

The basic physiological fact of weight loss and weight gain can be broken down into two simple basic factors:

1. The number of calories that you consume (food/combustible material).
2. The amount of time that you walk (energy output/calories burned).

These two simple basic facts are all you need to know regarding weight loss. If you restrict the number of **calories** that you eat you will **lose weight**. And, if you **walk** more you will **lose weight**.

CALORIES CONSUMED VS. CALORIES BURNED

The key to success in **THE WEIGHT-LOSS WALKING PROGRAM** is that you don't have to diet to lose or to maintain your weight.

How many of us have noticed that after we return from a vacation we are surprised to see that we have gained little or no weight? This is because we walk two to three times as much on a vacation as we do at home. Therefore, even though we eat richer, higher calorie foods on our vacation, our weight stays pretty much the same. **Walking burns calories** from the excess food that we eat. This is the principle behind **THE WEIGHT-LOSS WALKING PROGRAM: WALKING BURNS CALORIES.**

For any successful diet program the secret ingredient is a reduction in the total amount of calories consumed. If, however, you do not limit your intake of calories you have no other alternative but to increase the energy expenditure (burning calories) in order to lose or maintain weight.

The equation, **"CALORIES CONSUMED VS. CALORIES BURNED"** is the basic formula for permanent weight loss.

With very little exception, most people are overweight because they either eat too much or exercise too little. Their food intake exceeds their energy expended. The result becomes an excess of fat stored in the body. For every **3,500** calories of excess food taken in we accumulate **one pound of fat.**

The biochemical process by which food is converted to energy or fat (potential energy) is called **METABOLISM,** and all of the food that you consume is either burned (oxidized) to meet the energy requirements of the body or it is stored for future use. The energy that we burn is used primarily for the vital functions of the internal organs (heart, lungs, brain, liver, nervous and endocrine systems) and the external work of the muscles of the body for walking, moving, lifting, talking. If your energy intake (food) is less than you need, then your body burns the stored energy that it has built up and you will lose weight. If the energy intake (food) is more than required, then the excess is stored in the body tissues in the form of fat and you gain weight.

EXERCISE AND CALORIES

Well, now I am sure you are saying, "I walk every day and I don't lose weight." Actually you do lose weight every time you walk; however, you gain it back by eating. Remember: **CALORIES TAKEN IN VS. ENERGY OUTPUT (CALORIES EXPENDED).**

Let's look at a few examples. The input of combustible material vs. energy output:

1. Steam engine
2. Auto engine
3. Coal furnace
4. Oil furnace

All of these examples have one common denominator, and that is the combustible material, in our case food, that is introduced into the machine (our body) which results in the production of energy (heat) and waste materials.

Weight control, weight maintenance, and physical fitness are functions of the utilization of energy in the body. It is simple to see, therefore, that if we control the input and output of energy, we can control our weight and physical fitness. The following three equations are the basic ingredients of **THE WEIGHT-LOSS WALKING PROGRAM.**

1. If food intake is less than energy output (walking), then stored food (fat) is burned to produce needed energy ⟶ you lose weight.
2. If food intake is more than energy output (walking), then excess energy is stored as fat in the tissues ⟶ you gain weight.
3. If food intake is equal to energy output (walking), then ⟶ your weight stays the *same*.

WHAT'S THE BEST WAY TO LOSE WEIGHT, CALORIE COUNTING OR EXERCISE?

Calorie reduction accounts for weight loss in only 20% of dieters. **Exercise**, however, with or without limiting calories is the sure road to weight reduction. According to the Health Insurance Institute in Washington, D.C., most obese people are not necessarily excessive eaters but they are significantly less active than their thinner companions. It is actually their **sedentary life** which accounts for the excess weight and this must be changed, either by a formal exercise program or by increasing the amount of physical activities, particularly walking, in their daily lives. A brisk walk for an hour a day could result in a 15 pound weight loss in a period of 6 months, providing the calorie intake remained the same.

In order to lose weight efficiently, the energy burned during exercise should actually come from the **body fat** and not from carbohydrates. After ½ hour of moderate exercise, only approximately ½ of the energy comes from carbohydrates while the remaining energy is taken from the body fats. Therefore, it is obvious that longer periods of exercise are better for weight reduction than brief bouts of strenuous exercise such as jogging. **Walking**, therefore, fits the bill perfectly since it is a moderate, low intensity exercise that can be continued for a longer period of time with less stress and strain on the heart. Therefore, we see that by increasing the time of the exercise from ½ to 1 hour we are able to utilize the energy from body fats rather than from carbohydrates, resulting in more complete weight control. In other words, you will maintain your weight-loss better by an **hour of walking** every day than by 30 minutes of jogging, even though both activities burn approximately the same number of calories.

THE WEIGHT CONTROL PRINCIPLE

In simple mathematics, in a **pound of body fat** there are approximately **3,500 calories**. Consequently, when you eat 3,500 more calories than your body actually needs, it stores up that pound, and when you take in 3,500 calories less than your body needs, you will lose a pound. It does not make any difference how long it takes your body to either store or expend this 3,500 calories. The final result always is that you either become fatter or thinner by one pound. This imbalance can take place over a day, a week, a month, or a year.

Following the same basic principle, we see that in order to begin a reducing diet you do not have to do anything except walk. It sounds simple but it is an actual fact. If you walk for **one hour every day,** you will burn up approximately **350 calories.** If you walk **one hour a day for 10 days,** then you will burn up **3,500 calories.** Therefore, when you burn up 3,500 calories by walking, you will lose a pound of body fat. It makes no difference how long it takes you to burn off these 3,500 calories, the end result is the same: You will actually **lose one pound of body fat.**

In elementary physics we learn that to move a given weight a distance of one foot requires the same amount of energy, whether you move the object quickly or slowly. The same principle applies with walking, with some minor exceptions. It is actually the **distance** that you travel in walking that is significantly more important than the speed at which you walk. Therefore, the calories that you burn depend upon the distance that you travel and not on the speed. An example is that if you run fast for 4 miles you will actually burn up only 10% more calories than you do by walking the same distance.

Overweight does not come overnight. Excess weight develops slowly; **no one ever became fat all of a sudden.** The gradual accumulation of extra calories that you store up day by day is the basis for excess body weight. For example, if you eat only 100 calories more per day than your body needs, then you will gain a pound every month. Likewise, if you eat approximately 100 calories less per day, you will lose a pound a month.

If you walk about 20 minutes a day, you will burn up approximately that same 100 calories and will lose a pound a month, or 10 pounds a year. If you walk one hour a day, you will burn up approximately 350 calories per day and lose 1 pound every ten days, or 3 pounds a month, or 36 pounds a year.

How many of us are willing to make the lifetime concession of being hungry on a forever diet? Most of us are not, and that is the basis for the failure of every diet perpetrated on the American public. However, if we continue on a **lifetime walking program,** then we will have a regular exercise that will control our weight for the rest of our lives. So, let's **walk** as if our **lives** and our **figures** depended on it. They do!

WALKING EXPENDS ENERGY (Burns Calories)

Walking actually **burns calories.** The following chart can give you an idea as to the energy expended in walking, which is actually the number of calories burned per hour.

One reason we find that fat tends to accumulate as we get older is because our physical activity tends to decrease while our food intake stays the same. It takes approximately 3,500 calories to either gain or lose one pound.

--------------------- TABLE I ---------------------

Walking Pace	Calories/ Minute	Calories/ Hour
Slow pace (2 mph)	4–5	240–300
Moderate pace (3 mph)	5–6	300–360
Fast pace (4 mph)	6–7	360–420

It becomes readily apparent that a one-hour walk at the **moderate pace** will burn up between 300–360 calories per hour. For example, if you take a **one-hour walk every other day** or a ½-hour walk daily, you will burn up approximately 1,225 calories per week (3½ hrs./wk. × approximately 350 calories per hour = 1,225 calories per week) or an average loss of **175 calories every day.**

THE WEIGHT-LOSS WALKING PROGRAM

THE WEIGHT-LOSS WALKING PROGRAM is based on a moderate walking pace (3 mph)—**TABLE I,** providing that there is *no change* in your daily intake of food. In other words, this weight-loss program is based upon **calories burned by walking only.** With **THE WEIGHT-LOSS WALKING PROGRAM,** you will lose weight without any changes or alterations in your daily diet. You are actually *walking off weight!*

The **moderate pace (3 mph)** is actually the ideal rate of walking for **THE WEIGHT-LOSS WALKING PROGRAM.** Three miles per hour is the speed that most of us use in everyday *brisk walking.* It can be carried on for long periods of time without undue stress and strain and is unlikely to cause excess fatigue. This schedule has been devised for maximum efficiency and weight loss. This walking schedule can easily fit into your daily routine no matter how busy your life is. It can be done almost anywhere, any time, any place, without special clothing or costly health club dues.

THE WEIGHT-LOSS WALKING PLANS

1. SLOW WEIGHT-LOSS WALKING PLAN

The slow weight-loss walking program is based on **a one-hour walk every other day** or a ½-hour walk every day. Walking at the moderate pace rate of 3 mph, you will burn up approximately **350 calories every hour** that you walk. Since it takes 10 hours of walking to burn up 3,500 calories, you will **lose one pound every 20 days** (a loss of 175 calories daily), using this walking program (175 calories per day × 20 days = 3,500 calories). For example, **walk:**

a) ½ hour daily × 350 calories/hour = 175 calories lost per day,

b) 3½ hours per week × 350 calories/hour = 1,225 calories lost per week,

c) 10 hours every 20 days × 350 cal./hr. = 3,500 calories or one pound lost every 20 days.

This slow weight loss program will result in an approximate **18-pound weight loss in one year.** This occurs without any alteration in your daily diet whatsoever. You have actually **walked off 18 pounds!**

2. MODERATE WEIGHT-LOSS WALKING PLAN

Again, with no change in your everyday diet, you can lose one pound every 10 days by simply walking **one hour every day of the week.** This additional weight loss occurs at the same walking speed of 3 mph as noted above in the **Slow Weight-Loss Walking Plan.** The only difference is that you are now walking for one hour every day. You will be burning up **350 calories** every day on a **1 hour walk** at a pace of 3 mph.

As we have already noted, it takes 10 hours of walking at 3 mph to burn up 3,500 calories or one pound. Therefore, if you walk for an hour every day, you will lose **one pound every 10 days.** This will result in an approximate weight loss of **3 pounds every month** or **36 pounds in one year.** Remember, you can actually **walk off 36 pounds** every year.

3. MAINTENANCE WEIGHT-CONTROL WALKING PLAN

After you have walked off as much weight as you want to lose and are now satisfied with your present weight, then you are ready for your walking bonus snack. You can have an **extra 175-calorie bonus snack every day** without gaining one extra ounce. Remember, you will still be walking **one hour every other day** or ½

hour daily on the **Slow Weight-Loss Walking Plan.** You will, therefore, be burning up 1,225 calories every week or 175 calories daily (3½ hours walking per week × 350 calories per hour = 1,225 calories per week or 175 calories every day).

Your ideal body weight will remain stable forever, providing you continue your **½ hour daily walk** or your **one hour every other day walk.** Think of it, a **175 calorie snack** (any snack) every day, in addition to your regular maintenance diet, without gaining an ounce.

Remember, these three weight-loss walking plans are based on **weight loss by walking only.** There is no change in your present diet. You will lose weight by walking only, providing you don't increase your current daily intake of calories. On the following chart, record the time and the approximate distance that you walk each day. Record your weight in the last column every Wednesday morning. Do not weigh yourself more often than once a week.

THE WEIGHT-LOSS WALKING PROGRAM
YOUR WEIGHT-LOSS WALKING RECORD

Week		Mon.	Tues.	Wed.	Thurs.	Fri.	Sat.	Sun.	Wed. AM Weight
1	Time								
	Distance								
2	Time								
	Distance								
3	Time								
	Distance								
4	Time								
	Distance								
5	Time								
	Distance								
6	Time								
	Distance								
7	Time								
	Distance								
8	Time								
	Distance								

2

SO YOU WANT TO LOSE WEIGHT FASTER!

HOW CAN I LOSE WEIGHT FASTER?

Dieting has developed into a billion-dollar business in the United States, since obesity is one of the major health conditions that affects nearly 70 million Americans. There are always new diet books, weight loss gimmicks, and fad diets that claim fast results in the weight reduction game. The majority of these have two things in common—they avoid the *nutritional requirements* and the *health* of the dieter. Any diet that restricts one or more food groups while advocating increased amounts of another, is nutritionally unsound. These so-called **fad diets** may, in fact, actually be hazardous to your health.

There is no such thing as a *miracle diet*. Crash diets which result in rapid weight loss usually are followed by what is known as the **rebound phenomenon.** This means that you may regain more weight than you actually lost during the diet. Weight is usually gained over a long period of time and cannot be lost in a few days or weeks. Many of my patients have been on a "forever diet," and have lost and re-gained enough weight to equal another whole person. The key to successful weight loss is a diet which provides the body with the **essential nutrients** and one that provides the dieter with a sound basis for a change in *lifetime eating habits.* Successful weight reduction, in addition to **burning calories** (walking), depends on **reducing the calories** from all of the basic food groups rather than concentrating on one or more foods. This combination of walking and calorie reduction is the basis for **THE DOCTOR'S WALKING DIET.**

It is not only necessary to be aware of the total number of calories that you consume daily, but it is equally important to be aware of the nutritional content of the various foods that you eat. By following the general rules outlined below, your diet will be properly balanced with the correct ratio of protein, carbohydrate, fat, minerals, and vitamins. This is essential for good nutrition.

The **U.S. Department of Agriculture and the Department of Health and Human Services** recently devised the dietary guidelines for Americans. These guidelines are:

1. Maintain ideal weight.
2. Eat a variety of foods.
3. Avoid too much sugar.
4. Avoid too much sodium (salt).
5. Avoid alcohol.
6. Avoid too much fat, especially saturated fat and cholesterol.
7. Eat foods with adequate starch and fiber content (fresh fruits, vegetables and whole-grain foods).
8. Avoid most processed snack foods.
9. Eat more fish and poultry, and less red meat.
10. Use low-fat dairy products.

For those of you who are now saying, "I can't wait 6 months to lose weight, I have a wedding in three weeks and I have to get into last year's dress," I have the answer to your prayers—**THE DOCTOR'S WALKING DIET!**

THE DOCTOR'S WALKING DIET combines all the weight-loss properties of **THE WEIGHT-LOSS WALKING PROGRAM** (Chapter 1), with the simple **reduction of calories** from your daily diet. This combination of walking plus calorie reduction results in **rapid, safe, effective weight loss.**

THE EFFECT OF EXERCISE ON APPETITE

Contrary to popular belief, exercise does not increase the appetite: It has an **appetite-depressing effect.** The following reasons have been given by researchers for this appetite suppressing effect of exercise:

1. Exercise controls the **brain center** (Appestat) which regulates the appetite. Increased exercise ⟶ decreased appetite.
2. The **blood flow** during and after exercise is directed away from the digestive tract toward the muscles engaged in exercise.
3. The **blood fats** are utilized as a source of energy instead of blood sugar during exercise.

Since blood sugar is the primary source of energy for the brain, a *low blood sugar* level can make you feel hungry. However, when we exercise, fat is released into the blood stream and it is utilized as a fuel to produce energy instead of the body using blood sugar. This enables the blood sugar to remain relatively constant and therefore you will not feel hungry since the body is *burning fat* rather than utilizing sugar as its source of energy.

These chemical changes which occur during exercise and immediately following exercise are especially important to the dieter, since you may engage in your walking diet program ½ to 1 hour prior to mealtime and subsequently experience a *decrease in your appetite*. Inactivity, on the other hand, stimulates the appetite control center and makes you hungrier.

THE DOCTOR'S WALKING DIET

Scientific research has shown that **exercise,** along with **calorie reduction,** is essential for the maintenance of any long-term diet program. Population studies have shown that individuals with sedentary jobs have more trouble maintaining their weight than people who were involved in active jobs. In general, healthy people as well as people with chronic diseases such as high blood pressure, heart disease, diabetes, and obesity will benefit from a program of *regular exercise* combined with a *low-calorie diet*.

Remember that in order to gain one pound of body weight you must take in 3,500 calories over any given period of time. In order to lose one pound of weight, we must either reduce the intake of calories by 3,500 calories or increase the amount of exercise (walking) that we do in our daily lives in order to burn up or expend the same 3,500 calories. Either a **reduction of calories eaten** or an **increased expenditure of calories burned (walking)** will result in the **same one-pound weight loss.**

The following **3 weight loss plans** will allow you to lose weight quickly, safely and easily without rebound weight gain. They include:

1. **THE DOCTOR'S WALKING DIET:**
   for fast, safe, effective, permanent weight loss,

utilizing a simple 3-step program, combining walking and calorie reduction.

2. **THE DOCTOR'S SPECIAL WALKING DIET:** with the built-in cheating factor, for those of us who can't resist temptation.

3. **THE DOCTOR'S F*A*S*T* 3-DAY DIET-WALK®:**

    offers the only complete **lifetime walking-diet** program **without calorie counting,** for permanent *weight control, health maintenance,* and *longevity* (discussed completely in Chapters 3 and 4).

1. THE DOCTOR'S WALKING DIET

STEP 1: WEIGHT LOSS BY WALKING

Let's review how easy it is to lose weight without reducing calories on the **Weight-Loss Walking Program** (Chapter 1).

1. **Slow Weight-Loss Walking Plan**
    a. Walk **one hour** every other day or **½ hour** daily.
    b. You burn up **175 calories** every day.
    c. You lose **one pound** every **20 days** or **18 lbs.** in **one year.**
2. **Moderate Weight-Loss Walking Plan**
    a. Walk **one hour** every day.
    b. You burn up **350 calories** daily.
    c. You lose **one pound** every **10 days** or **36 lbs.** in **one year.**

STEP 2: WEIGHT-LOSS BY CALORIE REDUCTION

Now let's see how you can lose an additional ½ lb., 1 lb., or 2 lbs. every week by simply reducing the number of calories from your diet each day **(Table II).**

How to Use Table II

1. Find your **PRESENT WEIGHT** on the 1st column of **TABLE II.** The 2nd column shows the number of calories you consume daily to maintain your present weight.
2. Follow the line across from the number of calories consumed daily to maintain your present weight and the next 3 columns show the number of calories you will have to consume daily if you desire to lose either ½ lb., 1 lb. or 2 additional lbs. per week.
3. What determines our weight, in addition to walking, is simply the **total number of calories** contained in the food that we eat. Since we have seen that it takes approximately 3,500 calories to lose one pound, it becomes obvious that by eliminating 500 calories daily (7 days × 500 calories = 3,500 calories) from our diet, we will lose one pound per week. In order to lose two pounds per week, we must reduce our daily caloric intake by 1,000 calories per day. It is unwise, however, from a health and nutritional standpoint, to consume less than 800–1,000 daily.
4. Consult **APPENDIX** for caloric values of various foods.

TABLE II
WEIGHT LOSS BY CALORIE REDUCTION

THE NUMBER OF CALORIES PER DAY NECESSARY TO:

PRESENT WEIGHT Present Weight	Maintain Present Weight	Lose ½ lb. per wk.	Lose 1 lb. per wk.	Lose 2 lbs. per wk.
Adult Females				
110	1,700	1,450	1,200	700
120	1,800	1,550	1,300	800
130	1,900	1,650	1,400	900
140	2,000	1,750	1,500	1,000
150	2,100	1,850	1,600	1,100
160	2,300	2,050	1,800	1,300
170	2,400	2,150	1,900	1,400
180	2,500	2,250	2,000	1,500
190	2,600	2,350	2,100	1,600
200	2,700	2,450	2,200	1,700

Adult Males				
130	2,300	2,050	1,800	1,300
140	2,400	2,150	1,900	1,400
150	2,500	2,250	2,000	1,500
160	2,700	2,450	2,200	1,700
170	2,800	2,550	2,300	1,800
180	2,900	2,650	2,400	1,900
190	3,100	2,850	2,600	2,100
200	3,200	2,950	2,700	2,200
210	3,300	3,050	2,800	2,300
220	3,400	3,150	2,900	2,400

STEP 3: WALKING & CALORIE REDUCTION COMBO

Now by combining the **Walking Weight-Loss Plans** (either ½ hour daily or 1 hour daily) with the simple reduction of calories, you have the basic fundamentals of **THE DOCTOR'S WALKING DIET (TABLE III).**

HOW TO USE TABLE III

1. The 1st column is the **DISTANCE** you walk each day.
2. The 2nd column is the number of **calories burned walking** each day.
3. The 3rd column is the number of **calories you must subtract** each day from your present diet, in order to lose 1, 5, 10, 15, or 20 lbs.
4. The 4th column is the **total calories** expended daily (calories burned walking and calories subtracted from diet).
5. The last columns indicate the **number of days** needed to lose 1, 5, 10, 15, or 20 lbs.
6. Consult **Appendix** for caloric values of different foods.

TABLE III
THE DOCTOR'S WALKING DIET
(½ HOUR DAILY WALK)

Miles Walked Daily	Calories Burned Walking	Minus Calories in Daily Diet	Total Calories Expended Daily	Days Needed to Lose:					Lbs.
				1	5	10	15	20	
1½ miles	175 cal.	0 cal.	175 cal.	20	100	200	300	400	days
1½ miles	175 cal.	175 cal.	350 cal.	10	50	100	150	200	days
1½ miles	175 cal.	325 cal.	500 cal.	7	35	70	105	140	days
1½ miles	175 cal.	525 cal.	700 cal.	5	25	50	75	100	days
1½ miles	175 cal.	700 cal.	875 cal.	4	20	40	60	80	days
1½ miles	175 cal.	1,000 cal.	1,175 cal.	3	15	30	45	60	days

(ONE HOUR DAILY WALK)

Miles Walked Daily	Calories Burned Walking	Minus Calories in Daily Diet	Total Calories Expended Daily	Days Needed to Lose:					Lbs.
				1	5	10	15	20	
3 miles	350 cal.	0 cal.	350 cal.	10	50	100	150	200	days
3 miles	350 cal.	150 cal.	500 cal.	7	35	70	105	140	days
3 miles	350 cal.	350 cal.	700 cal.	5	25	50	75	100	days
3 miles	350 cal.	525 cal.	875 cal.	4	20	40	60	80	days
3 miles	350 cal.	825 cal.	1,175 cal.	3	15	30	45	60	days
3 miles	350 cal.	1,400 cal.	1,750 cal.	2	10	20	30	40	days

2. THE DOCTOR'S SPECIAL WALKING DIET

We have many daily temptations such as a cone of ice cream, a slice of pizza or a cold beer, which at times can be very irresistible. With **THE DOCTOR'S SPECIAL WALKING DIET** you have a **built-in safety valve** that allows you to **cheat** occasionally. After indulging in your favorite snack food, consult the following table **(Table IV)** and walk the extra minutes noted to get rid of the extra calories you've picked up.

If you would just like to walk off that extra dessert, slice of pizza or drink that you had today, then the following list shows how many minutes of walking at the moderate pace (3 mph) are necessary to burn up the caloric value of those foods. This type of plan should only be used if your weight and calorie intake are stable. Remember, this plan is for cheating only, when temptation is too much for your willpower.

If your favorite snack food does not appear on the following list, you still can easily calculate the number of minutes you have to walk in order to burn off any food that you choose. Find out the number of calories for that particular food (consult **APPENDIX**) and divide by 6, and you will have the number of minutes it would take to walk it off. This formula is derived from the fact that walking at the moderate pace (3 mph) burns approximately 6 calories per minute.

TABLE IV
THE DOCTOR'S SPECIAL WALKING DIET
MINUTES WALKING (3 MPH) TO BURN CALORIES
(SNACK FOODS)

American cheese (1 sl.)	16 minutes
apple (medium)	15 minutes
bagel (1)	23 minutes
banana (medium)	16 minutes
beer (12 oz.)	30 minutes
bologna sandwich	50 minutes
cake (1 slice pound)	63 minutes
chocolate bar/nuts (1 oz.)	28 minutes
chocolate cookies (3)	25 minutes
doughnut (jelly)	40 minutes
frankfurter & roll	50 minutes
hamburger (4 oz.) and roll	73 minutes
ice cream sundae	75 minutes
milk shake, choc. (8 oz.)	42 minutes
muffin, blueberry	25 minutes
peanuts, in shell (2 oz.)	37 minutes
pie, apple (1 slice)	46 minutes
pizza (1 slice)	40 minutes
pretzel, soft (ex. Superpretzel®)	30 minutes
soda, cola type (12 oz.)	24 minutes
wine, white (4 oz.)	14 minutes
whiskey, rye (1 oz.)	17 minutes

A RECORD OF YOUR WALKING DIET

On the following chart you can record your progress on
THE DOCTOR'S WALKING DIET.

1. Record the **Time** and approximate **Distance**
walked each day.

2. Record the **Calories Burned Walking** and the
Calories Subtracted from your present diet. (Table II
shows how many calories you consume daily and Table
III illustrates calories burned walking.)

3. Then record the **Total Calories Expended Daily** which is the total of calories burned and calories subtracted.

4. Record your **weight** no more than once a week (don't be discouraged if your weight stays the same or occasionally goes up—this can be explained by fluid retention and metabolic changes).

5. **Total each column** at the end of each week (example: number of hrs. walked per week, distance walked per week, total calories expended and weight lost each week).

6. Remember that when the total calories expended column adds up to **3,500 calories** you will **lose one pound.** One pound is always lost when 3,500 calories are burned, no matter how long it takes.

7. **Weight loss** never proceeds in a straight line. In other words, even though you are following **THE DOCTOR'S WALKING DIET** your weight loss occasionally levels off or plateaus. This simply is a temporary metabolic re-adjustment that your body is making to the weight reduction. If you continue on the walking diet program without becoming discouraged, then your weight loss will again proceed after this temporary slow-down.

8. You may use either the ½ hour or 1 hour daily walking plan, or any combination of both plans for your walking diet record. If the weather is bad, remember to use the **Indoor Shape-Up/Slim-Down Program** (Chapter 11).

THE DOCTOR'S WALKING DIET
YOUR WALKING DIET RECORD

Week/Day	Time Walked	Miles Walked	Calories Burned Walking	Minus Calories From Present Diet	Total Calories Expended Daily	Weight Lost
(EXAMPLES:)	1 hour	3 miles	350 calories	+ 500 calories	= 850 calories	
	½ hour	1½ miles	175 calories	+ 0 calories	= 175 calories	
MON.						
TUES.						
WED.						
THURS.						
FRI.						
SAT.						
SUN.						
TOTAL WK. #1						
MON.						
TUES.						
WED.						
THURS.						
FRI.						
SAT.						
SUN.						
TOTAL WK. #2						

THE DOCTOR'S WALKING DIET
YOUR WALKING DIET RECORD

Week/Day	Time Walked	Miles Walked	Calories Burned Walking	Minus Calories From Present Diet	Total Calories Expended Daily	Weight Lost
(EXAMPLES:)	1 hour	3 miles	350 calories	+ 500 calories	= 850 calories	
	½ hour	1½ miles	175 calories	+ 0 calories	= 175 calories	
MON.						
TUES.						
WED.						
THURS.						
FRI.						
SAT.						
SUN.						
TOTAL WK. #3						
MON.						
TUES.						
WED.						
THURS.						
FRI.						
SAT.						
SUN.						
TOTAL WK. #4						

3

F*IRST A*MERICAN S*UPER DIET*

You have seen how easily you can lose weight on **The Weight-Loss Walking Program** (Chapter 1) by walking only, without any change whatsoever in your diet. And for those of you who want to lose weight faster, then **The Doctor's Walking Diet** (Chapter 2) will let you speed up your weight loss program. This diet utilizes a combination of walking and calorie reduction for safe, effective weight loss.

Chapters 3 and 4 describe the ultimate diet: The **DR.'S F*A*S*T* 3-DAY DIETWALK®**. Here at last is a diet program which is unique in the annals of dieting. There are no calories to count, no foods to weigh, no special menus to prepare, and no starvation tactics to endure. This fast and easy diet plan enables you to lose weight rapidly, stay thin, and keep trim for a lifetime. In addition to keeping you thin, the diet provides a built-in protective mechanism against many diseases and degenerative conditions of aging. The **DR.'S F*A*S*T* 3-DAY DIETWALK®** is designed to help you lose weight fast, stay thin, keep fit and live longer—all without calorie counting or gimmick diet plans.

FAD DIETS MAY BE HAZARDOUS TO YOUR HEALTH

Many weight-loss programs are based on non-medical principles and can be classified as "gimmicks" or "fad diets." They promise rapid sure-fire weight loss programs with no regard for the health of the dieter. Any diet that advocates an increased intake of one of the basic food groups at the expense of another is nutritionally unsound.

As strange as it sounds, all fad diets fall into two main categories: **LOW CARBOHYDRATE** and **LOW PROTEIN.** No matter which new diet comes out each spring or fall, they all are based on these two principles, regardless of the doctor, institution, or hospital that the diet is named after.

1. LOW CARBOHYDRATE DIETS (or high protein diets)

Low-carbohydrate diets are the most common form that most fad diets are based upon. They keep reappearing every year under a different name (water diets, drinking man's diets, rapid weight loss diets, bacon and eggs diets, eat all you want diets, high protein diets, etc.); however, they all are basically **low in carbohydrates** and **high in fat and protein.** If you check all the diet books in your favorite book store, you'll be surprised to see that at least two out of three of them are based on this low-carbohydrate principle.

These low-carbohydrate diets all have the same underlying defects: they are **nutritionally unsound,** they are **potentially hazardous** to your health, and they are **ineffective for permanent weight loss.** In fact, most people tend to gain more weight than they lost, once they stop the diet (rebound phenomenon).

These diets lead to a metabolic disorder known as

"KETOSIS" which is actually the same condition that occurs in diabetics. This condition can have the following possible **side effects:** general weakness, lack of stamina and strength, nausea and vomiting, dehydration, loss of calcium from the body, mental clouding and memory loss, muscle cramps and fainting. Other **more serious disorders** that have been infrequently reported are: kidney disorders and kidney failure in those people with underlying kidney disease; heart beat irregularities, heart attacks and strokes caused by the buildup of cholesterol in the arteries; and high blood pressure and vascular disease.

These diets produce rapid weight loss, which in turn produces **rapid weight gain** when the diet is stopped. For each gram of sugar stored in the body, **3 grams of water** are also stored. These diets cause the body to rapidly deplete itself of sugar, thus causing a rapid weight loss which is mostly water, not body fat. When the sugar reservoir runs out, the water loss stops and the weight loss levels off. Then the dieters rapidly regain their weight with some additional pounds to spare, after they become discouraged and resume normal eating habits.

2. LOW PROTEIN DIETS (or high carbohydrate diets)

Low protein diets are the next most common type of gimmick quick weight loss diets. They essentially all have the same basically unsound nutritional principles: **low in protein** and **high in carbohydrates and fat.** They are listed, again, under a variety of different names (grapefruit diets, fruit and enzyme diets, salad diets, vegetarian diets, cabbage diets, fasting diets, big city suburban diets, high carbohydrate diets, etc.), and usually **caution** the dieter against staying on the diet for too long a time because of possible side effects. Many of these diets also advocate periods of fasting.

The human body has **no mechanism for storing protein.** Weight loss which occurs from this type of diet results in the loss of **muscle tissue** as well as fat, which is a dangerous situation. When the weight is rapidly regained after stopping the diet, the lost muscle tissue is usually replaced with **fat.**

A protein deficient diet eventually results in the body literally consuming itself from within. Early in the course of the diet, the **hair** becomes fine and thin and loses its natural luster. Then the **nails** become brittle and cracked and slow their growth rate. Eventual loss of protein from the **skin, muscles** and **internal organs** results in easy bruising, muscle weakness and malfunction of the internal organs. These diets are usually **deficient in many essential vitamins and minerals** which may cause diarrhea and aggravate pre-existing stomach and intestinal problems.

3. LIQUID OR POWDERED PROTEIN DIETS

The most flagrant of the fad diets are the ones that promote the use of powdered or liquid protein combined with vitamin and mineral concentrates. These products are used in conjunction with total or partial **fasting** diet regimens. These diets crop up from year to year with different, fancy, impressive titles claiming that theirs is the ultimate diet plan. In recent years we have had a flood of liquid and powdered protein diets, many of which caused **heart irregularities** and, rarely, cardiac deaths. Other serious side effects include: improper nitrogen balance, potassium depletion, kidney disorders and the development of gout from high blood uric acid. The AMA has recently recommended a warning label for these protein products. I would never recommend this type of diet for any of my patients, nor, I am sure, would any of my colleagues. Man cannot live by powder or liquid concentrate alone!

4. STARCH BLOCKERS

The latest entry to the gimmick-fad diet field are the so-called "starch blockers." These tablets allegedly block starch digestion and thus promote weight loss. There is new evidence presented to the Food & Drug Administration indicating that these starch blockers are worthless and potentially hazardous. The FDA has recently ruled that these tablets are drugs and not food products and therefore need testing before they can be marketed. The sale of these products has recently been banned by the FDA; however, many pharmacies and health food stores continue to sell these products.

There have been numerous medical studies, including a recent report in the *New England Journal of Medicine* (12/21/82), that have found no evidence of blocked starch digestion or reduced calorie absorption. In other words, these tablets are virtually worthless as a weight-loss aid.

The FDA has also received many reports of side effects from these products, including nausea, vomiting, diarrhea, abdominal cramps and constipation. Other more serious reactions reported have included both liver and pancreas damage and one apparent death from an acute inflammation of the pancreas.

5. OVER-THE-COUNTER DIET PILLS

A report published in *Medical World News* (3/14/83) stated that high doses of *phenylpropanolamine* (PPA), a common ingredient in over-the-counter diet pills, may be associated with strokes and other serious disorders. This drug, which has amphetamine-like characteristics, may possibly be linked in some cases to the development of headaches, emotional disorders, high blood pressure, heart irregularities, kidney failure, convulsions and strokes.

The FDA has previously stated that PPA is safe for use as a weight control aid. However, in light of these recent findings, the Center for Science in the Public Interest wants the FDA to make PPA a prescription drug.

All of these fad diets and diet aids have two things in common: they are nutritionally unsound and they are potentially hazardous. The human body cannot survive indefinitely on these diets without serious side effects. Most fad diets also have what is called **"rebound phenomenon."** After the weight is initially lost, there is a plateau reached where no further weight is lost. The dieter, discouraged with the results, begins to eat because of depression and anxiety and actually gains more weight than was originally lost.

IS THERE REALLY A F*A*S*T*, EASY, SAFE, & EFFECTIVE DIET?

In addition to consuming food, Americans are consumed with the idea that the latest diet fad is the answer to their problem—the ultimate solution to endless pigging out. And so the dieter becomes an expert on the "new diet program" expounded by the latest book or TV talk show "diet expert." Then we begin our relentless search for alfalfa sprouts, seaweed, sunflower seeds, goat's milk, and other exotic and gourmet diet foods.

How many of us have the time, money or the energy to shop for special foods or the time to spend hours preparing low calorie gourmet meals? Perhaps for a few days, or at the most a few weeks, this type of diet planning and preparation can be interesting; however, as soon as you realize that it becomes tedious or time-consuming the diet is finished. Then of course it's back to the old way of preparing and eating meals—

what's **fast, easy** and **convenient.** Yes, any diet that takes us away from our daily routine is doomed to failure.

These arguments against diet programs in general is what prompted me to develop the **DR.'S F*A*S*T* 3-DAY DIETWALK®** for my patients. Diets that are based on quick weight-loss schemes are doomed to failure at the start. The reason is that although initially you can lose weight on a fad diet, it is almost impossible to continue the diet for a prolonged period of time. Consequently, what happens is the old "rebound phenomenon"—you gain the weight promptly back with some additional pounds to spare.

NO CALORIES TO COUNT!

How many of us have had the frustrating experience of working like mad to take off those extra pounds, only to have them reappear before we've had a chance to enjoy being thin? This rapid rebound weight gain is the basic shortcoming of most diet programs and the cause of countless hours of frustration and misery.

The **DOCTOR'S F*A*S*T* 3-DAY DIETWALK®** offers a permanent solution to this weight-loss, weight-gain cycle. This diet program provides the best of both worlds. It is an effective weight reduction program and an equally effective weight control program. Now at last here is a fast, safe method to lose weight and stay thin permanently. This diet program offers the only effective weight control program **without counting calories.** This is starting to sound too good to be true. Well it is true! In fact, this program is the easiest, most effective weight loss and weight control program ever conceived.

Remember, this is the only diet program that you will need for the rest of your life. It is easy to remember, easy to follow and easy to maintain. There are *no calories to count,* foods to weigh or measure, diet charts to consult or complicated meals to prepare. Here at last is an effective program that provides permanent weight control without counting calories.

AT LAST, A DIET THAT'S GOOD FOR YOU TOO!

The **DR.'S F*A*S*T* 3-DAY DIETWALK®** is a medically sound, effective diet that I developed in conjunction with the **DOCTOR'S WALKING DIET** (Chapter 2). This diet not only insures **weight loss** and **weight maintenance,** but it is the only diet that is medically formulated for **good health.** In fact, this diet may prevent or slow the progress of many of the diseases that affect hundreds of thousands of Americans each year.

During the past five years I have intensively researched the medical and scientific literature in order to develop this particular "diet program" designed for *weight loss, health* and *fitness.* The concepts and ideas presented here are the compilation of thorough investigative study and research.

The 3-Day Diet program was formulated for my patients who, like you, were tired of counting calories or following gimmick diet plans. This diet program is truly easy, safe and effective. During the past 5 years over 2,500 of my patients have lost and maintained their weight safely and effectively on this easy-to-follow diet program.

This diet can be followed for a *lifetime,* and is the only diet that doesn't become boring since it is continually satisfying to the palate. It will work both as a **weight reduction** and a **weight maintenance** diet forever. And if that's not enough, remember it is the only diet proven to be good for your *health.* No other diet can make that claim! At last, a diet that's good for you too!

F*IRST A*MERICAN S*UPER DIET*

The **DR.'S F*A*S*T* 3-DAY DIETWALK®** is actually a **high fiber diet** combined with a diet that is **low in cholesterol, saturated fat, salt** and **sugar.** When combined with a regular **walking** program, it is the only diet that has been proven to be effective in both weight control and health maintenance.

The **high fiber** content of this diet provides a built-in mechanism against gaining weight and developing many diseases. By reducing the **saturated fat and cholesterol** content of the diet we eliminate many high fat calories that add extra weight and can clog up our arteries.

The **low sugar** content of the diet eliminates nutritionally deficient calories that add senseless pounds and may contribute to the development of heart disease and diabetes. Reducing the **salt** content prevents excess accumulation of fluids and may help to prevent hypertension in susceptible people.

Even the amount of **caffeine** is limited in this diet since excess amounts can stimulate the appetite center—the very thing we are trying to prevent. Excess caffeine can result in nervousness, insomnia, palpitations and headaches, and it may play an adverse role in certain breast, pancreas and heart disorders.

These factors are what makes the **DR.'S F*A*S*T* 3-DAY DIETWALK®** effective in weight control as well as in disease prevention. Finally you have a diet that is as good for the inside of you as it is for the outside. Here is a safe, effective diet program that can be continued for a lifetime, providing permanent *weight control, good health* and *physical fitness.*

The **DR.'S F*A*S*T* 3-DAY DIETWALK®** is—*easy* to remember, *easy* to follow and *easy* to maintain. No special foods to buy, no involved food preparation, no calories to count, no foods to weigh, no adding up grams, and no worrying about fat, protein and carbohydrate content of foods. The diet plan does all this automatically for you. *Simplicity* is the key ingredient that is missing from the majority of diet programs.

By my careful analysis of the foods included in the diet you are assured of obtaining a **balanced, nutritional diet** that is both beneficial to your health and slimming to your body. This diet program will not only guarantee you a trim, lean body for the rest of your life, but can, according to proven medical authorities, add years to your life by retarding, and in many cases preventing, the development of many of the diseases that affect all of us.

Chapters 4 and 5 will deal with the weight-loss and weight-control aspects of the **DOCTOR'S F*A*S*T* 3-DAY DIETWALK®**. Chapters 6, 7 and 8 will concentrate on the health benefits provided by this diet program. You will also see from a detailed analysis of the diet in these chapters how certain diseases and degenerative conditions may be prevented. As an added benefit, of course, you will remain *thin* and *trim* forever with an increased *vitality* and *energy* that you never knew existed within your body. This is the F*irst A*merican S*uper dieT* that will keep you *thin, healthy* and *fit,* and will add years to your life.

TWELVE REASONS WHY THIS DIET IS CALLED THE F*IRST A*MERICAN S*UPER DIET*

What type of diet is it?

1. F*ast A*nd S*imple weight-loss dieT*
2. F*ast A*nd S*afe walking dieT*
3. F*ast A*nd S*ure weight-control dieT*

How does it work?

4. F*iber A*nd low S*aturated fat & cholesterol dieT*
5. F*iber A*nd low S*alt dieT*
6. F*iber A*nd low S*ugar dieT*

Are there any other benefits?

7. F*irst A*nti-aging S*uper dieT*
8. F*irst A*nti-cancer S*uper dieT*
9. F*irst A*nti-disease S*uper dieT*

What else does it do?

10. F*itness A*nd S*lim-down dieT*
11. F*itness A*nd S*hape-up dieT*
12. F*itness A*nd S*imple exercise dieT*

How much weight will you lose and how long will it take? How long and how far do you have to walk? The answers to these and other questions can be found in the next chapter, for those of you who can't wait to get on the F*A*S*T* track!

4

THE DOCTOR'S F*A*S*T* 3-DAY DIETWALK®

THE DOCTOR'S F*A*S*T* 3-DAY DIETWALK® MEAL PLANS

The following diet was named the F*A*S*T* 3-DAY DIETWALK® because it is a F*ast A*nd S*imple dieT*. The diet is divided into the following **3 diet-day meal plans:**

MONDAY & THURSDAY   MEAL PLAN #1
TUESDAY & FRIDAY   MEAL PLAN #2
WEDNESDAY & SATURDAY   MEAL PLAN #3
SUNDAY   FREE DAY

In other words, Monday and Thursday are the same meal plan, Tuesday and Friday are the same, as are Wednesday and Saturday. Sunday is essentially a **FREE DAY.**

Once you've completed the first week, the **DR.'S F*A*S*T* 3-DAY DIETWALK®** will become an automatic part of your everyday schedule. The simplicity inherent in the diet is profound. There is no need to

54

remember what to eat at home or what to order in a restaurant for any particular meal. The diet consists of only 3 diet meal plans each week.

Won't this type of diet become monotonous? Definitely not! There is such a variety of foods included in this diet that your taste buds will never tire of this healthful, nutritional, palatable diet program. By varying the nutrients in the diet, there are never hunger pangs or food cravings.

Remember, the **DR.'S F*A*S*T* 3-DAY DIET-WALK®** is the only diet that in addition to controlling weight, will add years to your life by providing essential, healthful **nutrients** and eliminating harmful components. This is a diet for *fitness* and *health* as well as *weight loss* and *weight-control*.

After you have reached your ideal weight on this fast 3 day diet program, you will never again have to worry about rebound weight gain. The **3-DAY MAINTENANCE DIETWALK®** plan enables you to stay thin, trim and fit utilizing a simple 3 day maintenance diet program discussed at the end of this chapter.

The amount of time that you walk each day is determined by how much weight you want to lose each week. Turn to the end of this chapter (Table V) to decide how many minutes you should walk daily to lose weight: fast, faster, fastest.

MONDAY & THURSDAY
Meal Plan #1

BREAKFAST:

1   whole medium orange or 4 oz. (½ cup) fresh or
    unsweetened orange juice
1   slice whole or cracked wheat bread
    (½ teaspoon whipped/diet margarine or 1 tsp.
    jelly)
1   cup coffee or tea
    (artificial sweetener & non-fat milk)

LUNCH:

1   cup/bowl soup (vegetable, tomato, lentil, bean,
    pea, celery, minestrone, consomme, chicken
    noodle/rice, Manhattan clam chowder—no
    creamed or pureed soups) and 2–3 whole wheat
    crackers
1   tossed salad with lettuce, tomato and cucumber
    (lemon and/or vinegar or 1 tsp. low-cal dressing)
1   cup coffee, or tea with artificial sweetener and
    non-fat milk, or diet soda

DINNER:

1   LT/4C salad (lettuce, tomato, celery, carrot,
    cucumber, cauliflower)
3–4 oz. lean beef pattie (broiled)
1   medium baked potato, including skin (no butter,
    margarine or sour cream)
1   cup decaffeinated (coffee, tea or diet soda)

MID-EVENING SNACK:

2   cups unbuttered, unsalted popcorn
      (hot air popcorn popper without oil)
1   glass decaffeinated (diet soda, coffee or tea)

BED-TIME SNACK:

¾–1 oz. cooked or cold whole grain (bran-type) un-
      sweetened cereal with cup non-fat milk, me-
      dium banana or 2 dozen raisins (½ oz.).

NUMBER OF MINUTES WALKING_____

TUESDAY & FRIDAY
Meal Plan #2

BREAKFAST:

½   medium grapefruit or 4 oz. (cup) fresh or un-
     sweetened grapefruit juice

1   bran, whole wheat or English muffin
     (½ teaspoon whipped/diet margarine or 1 tsp.
     jelly)

1   cup coffee or tea
     (artificial sweetener and non-fat milk)

LUNCH:

2–3 oz. (⅓–½ cup) tuna or chicken salad (1 tsp. mayon-
     naise), with lettuce, tomato and ⅓ cup coleslaw;
     and 2–3 whole wheat crackers

1   cup coffee or tea with artificial sweetener and non-
     fat milk, or diet soda

DINNER:

1   LT/4C salad (lettuce, tomato, celery, carrot,
     cucumber, cauliflower)

3–4 oz. baked or broiled fish (flounder, haddock,
     halibut, cod, sole, bass, bluefish, perch, trout)
     with lemon

½   cup broccoli, Brussels sprouts, carrots, zucchini,
     squash, cauliflower, spinach or green beans—no
     added butter (choose any two)

1   cup decaffeinated (coffee, tea or diet soda)

MID-EVENING SNACK:

1–2 med. unsalted hard pretzels (Old Fashion/Dutch
      type)
1   glass decaffeinated (diet soda, coffee or tea)

BED-TIME SNACK:

½–¾ cup low-fat vanilla yogurt or low-fat cottage
      cheese with 2 tsp. wheat germ or miller's bran

NUMBER OF MINUTES WALKING_____

WEDNESDAY & SATURDAY
Meal Plan #3

BREAKFAST:

4   medium dried or stewed prunes (stewed in ar-
    tificial sweetener and water) or 2 oz. (¾ cup)
    prune juice
1   slice whole or cracked wheat bread
    (½ teaspoon whipped/diet margarine or 1 tsp.
    jelly)
1   cup coffee or tea
    (artificial sweetener and non-fat milk)

LUNCH:

½–¾ cup fresh fruit salad on bed of lettuce with ⅓–½
    cup low-fat cottage cheese and 2–3 whole wheat
    crackers
1   cup coffee or tea with artificial sweetener and non-
    fat milk, or diet soda

DINNER:

1   LT/4C salad (lettuce, tomato, celery, carrot,
    cucumber, cauliflower)
3–4 oz. broiled or baked chicken breast, skin removed
1   cup brown long whole grain rice; or ½ cup frozen
    or 1 small ear whole kernel corn (no butter,
    margarine, or salt)
1   cup decaffeinated (coffee, tea or diet soda)

MID-EVENING SNACK:

2   cups unbuttered, unsalted popcorn
        (hot air popcorn popper without oil)
1   glass decaffeinated (diet soda, coffee or tea)

BED-TIME SNACK:

1   small/medium piece fresh fruit (apple, pear, peach,
        plum, banana, apricot or nectarine); or ½ can-
        taloupe or melon with ¼–⅓ cup raspberries,
        strawberries or blueberries

NUMBER OF MINUTES WALKING_____

SUNDAY—FREE DAY

(1,500 calorie limit for females and 1,800 calorie
limit for males)
Sample Menus

BRUNCH:

½ cantaloupe or melon

1 bagel or English muffin (½ tsp. whipped or diet margarine, or 1 tsp. jelly)

1–2 oz. smoked fish with lettuce, tomato and onion

½–1 tsp. cream cheese

2 cups coffee or tea (artificial sweetener & non-fat milk)

4 oz. orange or grapefruit juice

2 slices rye, pumpernickel or whole wheat bread (½ tsp. whipped or diet margarine, or 1 tsp. jelly)

1–2 eggs, any style (use Teflon pan) or vegetable spray—no butter or margarine

OR 1–2 slices bacon (lean)

2 cups coffee or tea (artificial sweetener & non-fat milk)

DINNER:

3–4 oz. steak (lean)

1 baked potato with skin (no butter or margarine)

½ cup of cooked vegetable of choice (no butter)

3–4 oz. veal, prepared any style (not breaded)

½ cup cooked spaghetti or pasta of choice with marinara or tomato sauce

OR 1 tbsp. parmesan cheese

1 LT/4C salad (lettuce, tomato, celery, carrot, cucumber, cauliflower)

8 oz. light beer

1 LT/4C salad (lettuce, tomato, celery, carrot, cucumber, cauliflower)

4 oz. light wine

EVENING SNACK:

½ cup mixed raisins and dry roasted unsalted peanuts

or

2 med. unsalted hard pretzels;

or 1 unsalted soft pretzel (Ex. Superpretzel®)

OR 1 baked apple (artificial sweetener and cinnamon and raisins

or

OR 1 portion mixed fresh fruit—⅔ cup (strawberries, blueberries, raspberries, grapes, sliced apples, pears, bananas, peaches, etc.); or 1 piece of fresh fruit

1 cup/glass decaffeinated (coffee, tea or diet soda)

REST

THE DR.'S F*A*S*T* 3-DAY DIETWALK® SUBSTITUTIONS

(The following substitutions can be made for any breakfast, lunch or dinner after you have completed 4 weeks on the F*A*S*T* 3-DAY DIETWALK®. Each substitution can be used only once in any given week.)

BREAKFAST:

¾–1 oz. cold whole grain cereal (bran-type) with any fresh fruit (½ cup) and ½ cup non-fat milk and artificial sweetener

or

¾–1 oz. cooked whole grain cereal with artificial sweetener, ½ cup non-fat milk, cinnamon and 2 dozen raisins (½ oz.)

or

2–4 oz. scrambled egg substitute (Ex. Egg Beaters®—FLEISCHMANN'S) with 1 slice rye or pumpernickel (½ tsp. whipped or diet margarine)

(Any of the above substitutions may have 1 cup coffee or tea with artificial sweetener and non-fat milk and 2 oz. (½ cup) fresh or unsweetened orange or grapefruit juice.)

LUNCH:

2 slices white-meat turkey or 2 slices low-fat cheese with lettuce, tomato on (1–2 slices) whole wheat bread (½ tsp. mayonnaise or mustard)

or

1 bacon (1–2 lean strips), lettuce and tomato sandwich on whole wheat bread (½ tsp. mayonnaise) and cup coleslaw

or

Small–medium chef salad with turkey and cheese only. Use lemon, vinegar or 1 tsp. of low-fat dressing

(Any of the above substitutions may have 1 cup coffee or tea with artificial sweetener and non-fat milk or 1 diet soda.)

DINNER:

Vegetable platter (broccoli, asparagus, squash, cauliflower, baked beans, carrots, green beans, spinach, mushrooms, stewed tomatoes); choose any three (½–¾ cup each); or 3–4 oz. baked eggplant or zucchini parmesan without oil, butter or breading

or

3–4 oz. veal tenders, baked with stewed tomatoes, onions, peppers and mushrooms, and 1 small baked potato, including skin (no butter, margarine or sour cream)

or

3–4 oz. roast turkey (white meat) with one small sweet potato (no butter or margarine) and cup of any green vegetable

(Any of the above substitutions may have 1 cup decaffeinated coffee, tea, or diet soda, and 1 LT/4C salad.)

F*AST A*ND S*IMPLE T*IPS

1. Follow the **DR.'s F*A*S*T* 3-DAY DIET-WALK®** menu plans exactly as outlined. The 1st approximate measurement of food listed in any meal is the amount for women, followed by the amount for men (Ex. 3–4 oz. or ½–¾ cup or cup/bowl, etc.). Measurements are approximate, not exact.

2. Substitutions are permitted only after the 4th week of the diet is completed.

3. You may use any breakfast, lunch or dinner substitution on any day of the week; however, you are only permitted to use that substitution once in any given week.

4. An 8 oz. glass of water should be taken ½ hour prior to each meal and again at bedtime. No in-between meal snacks are allowed. Salting of food not permitted.

5. **SUNDAY** is a free day on the **DR.'S F*A*S*T* 3-DAY DIETWALK®**, as long as you don't exceed 1,500 calories (female) or 1,800 calories (male). Several sample menus are listed as possible examples. Remember you can eat whatever you want on this free day as long as you stay under the calorie limit. Remember: **REST!** No walking required on Sunday.

6. You may add any combination of the following items to your dinner entree: tomatoes, zucchini, peppers (green or red), shallots, mushrooms or onions. These can be sauteed using a non-caloric vegetable spray only (Ex.: Pam®); or just broiled or baked along with the entree. Omit regular dinner vegetable.

7. Dinner **Monday** and **Thursday** (optional meal plan #1: lean beef pattie) can be eaten at any fast-food restaurant. Order ¼ lb. hamburger without roll and add all the fixings (once a week only).

8. Dinner **Tuesday** and **Friday** (optional meal plan #2: fish) can be steamed or poached with carrots, onions, peppers, tomatoes, mushrooms, or celery (once a week only). Omit regular dinner vegetable.

9. Dinner **Wednesday** and **Saturday** (optional meal plan #3: chicken) can be stir-fried in a wok (using vegetable spray, Ex.: Pam®) with snow peas, broccoli, carrots, bamboo shoots, water chestnuts, mushrooms, or onions (once a week only). Omit regular dinner vegetable.

10. You may have any of the following items: sugar-free decaffeinated soda, fresh lemon or lime juice (not reconstituted), artificial sweetener, seasonings and spices (except salt), decaffeinated coffee and tea, vinegar, herbs, club soda, bouillon and mineral or tap water.

11. Baking and broiling permitted when done on rack. You may boil or steam vegetables, meat, fish or poultry. Do not stew, fry or saute. Cook with seasonings, not salt or salt products.

12. Get in the habit of always asking for milk (preferably non-fat) when ordering coffee. Creamers (dairy & non-dairy) are high in saturated fat and calories.

13. One ounce of whole grain cold or hot cereal varies in portion size (Ex.: ½, ¾ cup, etc.) with each brand cereal. Always check the label to see how much of a cup of cereal equals 1 oz.

14. Limit caffeine to two cups coffee, tea or diet soda daily, since excess caffeine may make you nervous and can also increase your appetite. Make it a habit to order decaffeinated for your "2nd cup."

15. Decrease the amount of salt since it has a tendency to retain fluid and may mask actual body weight reduction. Salt also may cause or aggravate hypertension in susceptible people.

16. Do not diet if you are a child, teenager or pregnant. During the growth process or when nourishing a fetus, nutrients must not be restricted.

17. Always check with your physician before starting any diet program, especially if you have a medical problem.

HOW MUCH WEIGHT CAN YOU LOSE AND HOW LONG WILL IT TAKE?

By following **THE DR.'S F*A*S*T* 3-DAY DIET-WALK®** meal plan exactly as outlined in this chapter, you have a safe effective weight reduction or weight control program. The amount of weight that you lose will depend on the one variable in the diet—the **TIME** that you *walk* each day. The following chart (Table V) indicates the various times that you may decide to walk

----------------------------- TABLE V -----------------------------

THE DR.'S F*A*S*T* 3-DAY DIETWALK®

TIME WALKED OR PEDALED (Every Day Except Sunday)		APPROXIMATE AMOUNT OF WEIGHT YOU WILL LOSE EVERY:	
Walk (3 mph) (Minutes)	Stationary Bike (12 mph) (Minutes)	1 Week (Pounds)	4 Weeks (Pounds)
15	7½	2	8
30	15	2⅙	8⅔
45	22½	2⅓	9⅓
60	30	2½	10

Note: The above weight-loss pattern is variable depending on body build and individual metabolism.

each day of the week (except Sunday). The last 3 columns show how many pounds you will lose each week and each month. Remember, your **diet meal plan always stays the same.** Only the *time* you walk each day can be changed according to how much weight you want to lose. If the weather does not permit walking, then ride your stationary bike (Chapter 11) according to the calculated times **(Table V).**

THE DR.'S F*A*S*T* 3-DAY MAINTENANCE DIETWALK®

1. After you have reached your ideal weight, follow the F*A*S*T* 3-DAY DIETWALK® MEAL PLAN for only 3 days each week (*Monday, Tuesday & Wednesday*).
2. For the next 3 days of each week (*Thursday, Friday* and *Saturday*) follow the 3-DAY MAINTENANCE DIETWALK® high fiber, low cholesterol meal plans outlined at the end of this chapter. Remember, Sunday is your **free day.**

3. **Walk** 60 minutes **3 days** per week or 30 minutes every day except Sunday. Your weight will remain constant.

4. If the weather is bad, ride your stationary bike (Chapter 11).

5. If you have the urge to cheat, then turn to Chapter 2 (**The Dr.'s Special Walking Diet**) and walk off your favorite snack. How about a pizza?

6. Remember to eat high fiber, low cholesterol foods and avoid those foods that are high in sugar, salt and saturated fat. **THE 3-DAY MAINTENANCE DIETWALK® high fiber, low cholesterol** diet menus appear at the end of this chapter. Follow this maintenance diet for *Thursday, Friday* and *Saturday* each week.

3-Day Maintenance Dietwalk®
Diet Meal Plans
(THURSDAY, FRIDAY & SATURDAY)
(Females 1,500–2,000 calories)
(Males 2,000–2,700 calories)
Depending on Body Build

BASIC MEAL PLAN □ (2000 Cal)

BREAKFAST

1 Serving Milk	List 1
1 Serving Cereal	List 4
1 Serving	List 6
1 Serving Fruit	List 3
2 Servings Bread	List 4
3 Servings Fat	List 5
1 Serving	List 6

SAMPLE MENU I
1 cup CARNATION Instant Nonfat Milk
1 cup Shredded Wheat with
2 tsp sugar and
1 small banana
2 slices rye toast with
3 tsp margarine
Coffee or tea

SAMPLE MENU II
1 cup CARNATION Instant Nonfat Milk
½ cup Farina with
2 tsp sugar and
1 cup strawberries
2 slices wheat toast with
3 tsp margarine
Coffee or tea

LUNCH

1 Serving Fruit	List 3
1 Serving Veg	List 3
1 Serving Veg	List 3
2 Servings Fat	List 5
1 Serving Meat	List 2
2 Servings Bread	List 4
1 Serving Milk	List 1

SAMPLE MENU I
½ cup orange juice
1 cup coleslaw with
¼ cup shredded carrot and
2 tsp salad dressing
⅔ cup lowfat cottage cheese
1 large whole wheat roll
1 cup CARNATION Instant Nonfat Milk

SAMPLE MENU II
½ cup apple juice
1 cup raw spinach with
½ cup raw mushrooms and
2 tsp salad dressing
2 oz Mozzarella cheese
6 rye wafers
1 cup CARNATION Instant Nonfat Milk

DINNER

1 Serving Veg	List 3
1 Serving Veg	List 3
2 Servings Fat	List 5
2 Servings Meat	List 2
1 Serving Veg	List 3
2 Servings Veg	List 3
1 Serving Fruit	List 3
1 Serving	List 6

SAMPLE MENU I

1 cup Romaine lettuce with
1 tomato and
2 tsp salad dressing
4 oz lemon-broiled halibut
1 small baked potato
1 cup steamed broccoli
1 fresh apple
Coffee or tea

SAMPLE MENU II

1 cup watercress with
¼ cup cooked beets and
2 tsp salad dressing
4 oz BBQ chicken
½ cup brown rice
1 cup steamed Brussels sprouts
small fruit salad
Coffee or tea

BEDTIME

1 Serving Milk	List 1
1 Serving Fruit	List 3

SAMPLE MENU I
1 package CARNATION Instant Breakfast with
Nonfat Milk
12 fresh grapes

SAMPLE MENU II
1 package CARNATION Instant Breakfast with
Nonfat Milk
1 fresh peach

WALK:
60 MINUTES 3 DAYS PER WEEK
or
30 MINUTES DAILY EXCEPT SUNDAY

SPECIAL INSTRUCTIONS

ALTERNATE MEAL PLAN □ (2700 CAL)

Follow 2000 Cal Basic Meal Plan and add through the
day:

1 Serving Meat	List 2
3 Servings Fruits or Vegetables	List 3
4 Servings Bread or Cereal	List 4
3 tsp Fat	List 5

FOR WEIGHT CONTROL:
Use the following Basic Meal Plans:

☐ **1800 Calories:**

3 Servings CARNATION Instant Nonfat Milk	List 1
3 Servings Meat	List 2
7 Servings Fruits or Vegetables	List 3
6 Servings Bread or Cereals	List 4
6 tsp Fat	List 5

☐ **1500 Calories:**

3 Servings CARNATION Instant Nonfat Milk	List 1
2 Servings Meat	List 2
7 Servings Fruits or Vegetables	List 3
5 Servings Bread or Cereals	List 4
5 tsp Fat	List 5

☐ **1200 Calories:**

2 Servings CARNATION Instant Nonfat Milk	List 1
2 Servings Meat	List 2
5 Servings Fruits or Vegetables	List 3
4 Servings Bread or Cereals	List 4
4 tsp Fat	List 5

☐ **1000 Calories:**

2 Servings CARNATION Instant Nonfat Milk	List 1
2 Servings Meat	List 2
3 Servings Fruits or Vegetables	List 3
3 Servings Bread or Cereals	List 4
4 tsp Fat	List 5

Reprinted with permission of Carnation Healthcare Services, Los Angeles, California. Adapted from Carnation Special Patient Diet Plans (Hyperlipoproteinemia Diet Plan).

3-DAY MAINTENANCE DIETWALK®
SUBSTITUTION LISTS
(THURSDAY, FRIDAY & SATURDAY)

LIST 1: MILK GROUP

Recommended:
Milk products which are low in dairy fats:
Fortified skimmed (nonfat milk).
Fortified lowfat milk.
CARNATION Instant Nonfat Milk.
Buttermilk.
Lowfat yogurt.
CARNATION Instant Breakfast.
CARNATION Evaporated Skimmed Milk.

SUBSTITUTION LISTS

*Cheeses made from skimmed or partially skimmed milk such as:
Cottage cheese.
Farmer's cheese.
Baker's cheese.
Hoop cheese.
Mozzarella cheese.
Sapsago cheese.
Processed modified-fat cheeses (skimmed milk and polyunsaturated fat).

Avoid or use sparingly:
Whole milk and whole milk products:
Chocolate milk.
Canned whole milk.
Ice cream.
All creams, including: sour, half and half, whipped.
Whole-milk yogurt.
Non-dairy cream substitutes (use only in coffee, not as a milk substitute).

Cheeses made from cream or whole milk.
Butter.

Amount recommended:
At least two 8-fl.-oz. cups per day.
1 serving = 8-fl.-oz. cup for milks, 1-oz. for hard cheeses, or ½ cup for CARNATION Instant Breakfast and CARNATION Evaporated Skimmed Milk.

*Cheeses may be substituted for the meat group. 1 oz. cheese = 1 oz. meat.

LIST 2: MEAT GROUP

Recommended:
In most meals: chicken, turkey, veal, fish, cheeses (see List 1, Milk Group). Less frequently: beef, lamb, pork, ham. Choose lean cuts of meat. Trim all visible fat before cooking. Bake, broil, roast, or stew.

Nuts and dried beans and peas:
These are high in vegetable protein and may be used occasionally in place of meat.
Avoid or use sparingly: Duck, goose. Shrimp and heart are high in cholesterol, so use no more than once a week.

Organ meats: Liver, kidney and sweetbreads are very high in cholesterol.
Egg yolks: Limit to 3 per week eggs as such and other foods containing egg yolks, such as cakes, batters, and sauces.

Amount recommended:
The equivalent of 2 servings daily. Count as a serving: 2 to 3 ounces of lean cooked meat, poultry, or fish—all without bones;
2 eggs;
1 cup dry beans, dry peas, or lentils;
4 tablespoons peanut butter.

LIST 3: VEGETABLE—FRUIT GROUP

Recommended: One serving should be a source of vitamin C: Broccoli, cabbage (raw), tomatoes, berries, cantaloupe, grapefruit, mango, lemon, orange, papaya, strawberries.

One serving should be a source of vitamin A: Broccoli, carrots, chard, chicory, escarole, greens, kale, peas, spinach, string beans, sweet potatoes, yams, watercress, winter squash, apricots, cantaloupe, mango, papaya.

Avoid or use sparingly: If you must limit calories, use sparingly starchy vegetables such as: Potatoes, corn, or lima beans. One serving (½ cup) can be substituted for one serving of bread.

Amount recommended:
At least 4 servings daily.
1 serving: ½ cup cooked or 1 cup raw vegetables or fruit;
1 medium apple, orange, banana or potato;
½ medium grapefruit or cantaloupe.

LIST 4: BREAD—CEREAL GROUP

Recommended: Bread made with a minimum of saturated fat:
White enriched (including raisin bread), Whole wheat, English muffins, French bread, Italian bread, Oatmeal bread, Pumpernickel, Rye bread, Rye wafers.

Biscuits, muffins, and griddle cakes made with an allowed oil as shortening.
Cereal (hot and cold). Melba toast, Matzo, pretzels.
Pasta: macaroni, spaghetti, noodles (except egg noodles).
Rice.

Avoid or use sparingly:
Commercial butter rolls, biscuits, muffins, donuts, sweet rolls, cakes, crackers, egg bread, cheese bread.
Commercial mixes containing dried eggs and whole milk.

Amount recommended:
At least 4 servings daily.
1 serving:
1 slice bread,
1 cup dry cereal or ½ to ¾ cup cooked cereal, cornmeal, grits or rice.

LIST 5: FATS AND OILS

Recommended:
Margarine.*
Liquid oil shortenings.
Salad dressings and mayonnaise containing any of these polyunsaturated vegetable oils:

Corn,
Cottonseed,
Safflower,
Sesame seed,
Soybean, or
Sunflower oil.

Avoid or use sparingly:
Solid fats and shortenings:
Butter, lard.
Salt pork fat.
Meat fat.
Completely hydrogenated margarines and vegetable shortenings.

Products containing coconut oil, peanut oil, and olive oil may be used occasionally for flavor, but they are low in polyunsaturates.

Amount recommended:
Include about 2–4 tablespoons daily, depending on caloric allowance.

(*Use only a polyunsaturated fat margarine such as Fleischmann's)

LIST 6: DESSERTS, BEVERAGE, SNACKS AND CONDIMENTS:

Acceptable: non-caloric or low calorie foods:

Tea, coffee (no cream), cocoa powder, water ices, gelatin, fruit whip, puddings made with nonfat milk, low-calorie drinks, vinegar, mustard, ketchup, herbs, spices.

Use in moderation when calories or carbohydrates are restricted: High calorie foods:

Frozen or canned fruit with sugar added.
Jelly, jam.
Marmalade.
Honey.
Sugar candies.
Imitation ice cream.
Cakes, pies, cookies and puddings made with polyunsaturated fat.

Angel food cake.
Nuts (especially walnuts).
Peanut butter.
Bottled drinks.
Fruit drinks.
Ice milk.
Sherbet.
Wine.
Beer.
Hard liquor.

Avoid or use sparingly:

Cakes, pies, cookies, frozen cream pies, and other commercial dessert mixes.
Commercial fried food such as potato chips and other deep-fried snacks.
Whole milk puddings.
Ice cream.

Note: The acceptable foods on this list are low in saturated fatty acids and cholesterol. You may need to limit the portions of the foods on this list so that you do not exceed your calorie allowance for maintaining a desirable weight.

Moderation should be observed, especially in the use of alcoholic drinks, ice milk, sherbet, sweets and bottled drinks.

Reprinted with permission of Carnation Healthcare Services, Los Angeles, California. Adapted from Carnation Special Patient Diet Plans (Hyperlipoproteinemia Diet Plan).

THE DOCTOR'S F*A*S*T* 3-DAY DIETWALK®
YOUR WEIGHT-LOSS RECORD

Week	Time	Mon.	Tues.	Wed.	Thurs.	Fri.	Sat.	Sun.	Wed. AM Weight
1	Walked or Pedaled							REST	
2	Walked or Pedaled							REST	
3	Walked or Pedaled							REST	
4	Walked or Pedaled							REST	
5	Walked or Pedaled							REST	
6	Walked or Pedaled							REST	
7	Walked or Pedaled							REST	

5

GREAT DIET & NUTRITION TIPS

DIET & NUTRITION FALLACIES

1. **Calories don't count. False!** This is the first of the many fallacies that people use in the weight-loss business. On the contrary, calories do count in a weight-gain, weight-loss program. In order to gain or lose a pound of fat you must eat or not eat 3,500 more calories than you use up. The type of calories are not important in this particular fallacy, since it is the total number of calories involved in weight loss and weight gain.

2. **A crash diet** is an excellent way to begin a weight-loss program. **False!** This is probably the worst way to begin a diet program since crash diets, which are usually low in carbohydrates, produce rapid fluid loss. This fluid loss has nothing to do with the amount of liquid that we drink, and it is only reflecting a change in the body's ability to hold fluid. The fallacy is that fat is not coming off in this type of program, and, in fact, protein can be lost during a crash diet, which may be harmful to the kidneys. When these diets are abandoned weight is gained rapidly, usually in the form of

fat, and the dieter may wind up with more fat than he/she started with.

3. **Exercise is unimportant** in weight reduction and control. **False!** Nothing can be further from the truth. Regular physical exercise and activity is the key point in a long-term exercise maintenance program. Exercise not only burns calories, but has an appetite-regulating effect on the brain's appetite-control mechanism. Exercise also favorably affects the metabolism by lowering blood pressure, blood cholesterol, blood sugar and in general, contributing to good health.

4. **Eating more in the morning** will put on less weight than eating food in the evening. **False!** The body does not distinguish between time of day and calories consumed. There is practically no significant difference in the time of day or night that one eats food.

5. **Certain foods can burn up calories,** such as grapefruit. **False!** This is entirely erroneous. The digestion of food does consume some energy from the process of digestion, but there is no food that expends enough energy during digestion to promote weight loss.

6. **It is better to smoke than be fat. False!** The initial weight gained from decreasing or stopping smoking can always be lost by a diet and exercise program; however, the permanent lung, heart and artery damage done by smoking can never be undone.

7. **Toasting bread reduces its calorie count. False!** Toasting only changes the bread's texture and taste but does not burn away calories.

8. **It does not make any difference whether you eat slowly or quickly** as far as appetite or weight gain are concerned. **False!** Eating a meal slowly and chewing the food thoroughly gives the body metabolism a chance to regulate and reduce its appetite-regulating center in the brain. This subsequently can reduce the appetite and make you more satisfied with less food. Eating

rapidly does not cause overweight; however, since many overweight people tend to eat rapidly and do not give the appetite suppressing mechanism time to work, they eat more.

9. **Since meat is high in protein, it does not cause weight gain. False!** Protein, no matter what the source, contains 4 calories per gram. Carbohydrate also contains 4 calories per gram. Fat, however, contains 9 calories per gram, more than twice as many calories as a gram of protein or carbohydrate. Since any excessive calories above the body's basic metabolic requirements results in an increased storage of fat, eating meat not only can cause weight gain but can cause a greater proportion of fat being deposited in the body because of its high fat content. Therefore, meat not only gives 4 calories per gram for its protein content, but it also gives 9 calories per gram for its fat content. Therefore, the greater the percentage of fat in the meat, the higher the caloric value.

10. **Since protein is the most important nutritional requirement of the body, high protein diets are the most beneficial and the healthiest. False!** Protein is a very important part of the body and is necessary in the diet for providing the amino acids (building blocks) for cellular activity, tissue repair and general maintenance of the body. However, protein is not the only essential requirement of our bodies. Carbohydrates, fats, vitamins, minerals, essential fatty acids and calories are necessary to provide energy and the basic ingredients to work the body's physiological and biochemical machinery properly. Any diet that is weighted in favor of one item or another, for example, the high protein diet, is not a helpful or nutritious type diet.

11. **As long as you take a vitamin supplement every day, it doesn't matter what foods you eat or drink. False!** Vitamin supplements will not provide all the daily re-

quirements of protein, carbohydrates, minerals, amino acids and essential fatty acids that the body needs. This is a widespread misconception about nutrition and dieting. Many complications have been noted by people on very low calorie diets combined with protein-vitamin supplements, because of the inability of the body metabolism, particularly the kidneys and liver, to adjust to this type of diet.

12. **If I skip breakfast and lunch and just eat a large supper, I will lose weight. False!** No matter when the calories are consumed in a given 24 hour period the total end result is the same. The basic formula is: calories consumed vs. calories expended; whether you eat 400 calories 3 times a day or 1,200 calories at one meal, the body does not know the difference. In addition, skipping meals is not a healthful way to embark on a diet program, since the appetite becomes over-stimulated late in the day and you not only eat a large dinner but continuous snacks throughout the evening.

13. **If I eat or snack at bedtime, the food will not be digested properly and I will gain weight. False!** Again, the same principle exists as to the total calories consumed in any 24 hour period vs. the total calories expended. This is the basic formula needed for weight gain, weight loss, or weight maintenance. Eating at bedtime will not put any more weight on than eating any other time of day or night. Some people, however, may develop indigestion when they eat immediately before bedtime.

14. **Liver and red meat are essential in the diet because of their high content of iron. False!** While liver and red meat are excellent sources of iron as well as other nutrients including protein, vitamin A, niacin, and riboflavin, they also have a high content of saturated fats and are not a necessary part of any dietary program. There are many other foods, including green

leafy vegetables, chicken, turkey and fish which have adequate quantities of iron without the high saturated fat content.

A BAKER'S DOZEN GREAT DIET TIPS

1. **Eat more slowly** with each meal. This involves taking smaller, less frequent bites and chewing each mouthful for a longer period of time. Pause between each section of the meal.

2. If you are still hungry when you have finished your first portion, **wait at least fifteen minutes** to see whether or not you really want another portion. In most cases your appestat (the brain appetite control mechanism) will be more than satisfied at the end of that period of time and you will not need a second helping.

3. Also restrict your meals to one, or perhaps two, locations in your home for eating. If you have no regular place to eat, then you will find that you are eating in every room; however, when food is restricted to **one main dining area,** there will be less tendency to snack during the day.

4. Make sure you **leave the table** as soon as you are finished eating and spend **less time in the kitchen** or areas that have a tendency to remind one of eating.

5. Make sure that you do not place **serving dishes** on the table during a meal for there will be more of a tendency to take second and third helpings. Be sure that you **do not leave food out** where you can repeatedly see it during the day.

6. Never go to the market on an empty stomach; you will buy snack foods (carbohydrate cravings). Also make it a point not to eat while watching **television** or **reading** since you will eat more while not concentrating on your meal.

7. Remember not to start a weight reduction pro-

gram just prior to the **holiday season** or before **vacation time** since these are the most unsuccessful times to begin this type of project.

8. **Fried foods** should be avoided, since, even though you drain excess fat away, the fried foods still retain a large percentage of fat which adds to the calories. **Boiling, broiling, baking,** or **steaming** are the best techniques for preparing foods.

9. **Fat on poultry and meat:** Always trim away visible fat from meat and fowl before cooking and remove visible fat at the table when eating. The skin of the chicken contains 25% of the fat content of the chicken and will add tremendously to the calories. Canned fishes, such as tuna and salmon, should be packed in water or the oils drained away.

10. **Hot foods** such as soups, and foods that require a lot of **chewing** will leave you with a greater feeling of satisfaction because they take a longer time to swallow and absorb. Make sure you **leave the table** as soon as you finish eating.

11. Eat **salad greens** and **vegetables** before the main course since these will take the edge off your hunger for higher calorie meat, poultry and fish portions. The best salad dressing is none. Salad dressings are high in fats and calories. Use calorie-free herbs, spices, lemon, vinegar, or occasionally a small amount (1 tsp.) low-fat, low-calorie dressing. **Restaurant tip:** dip your fork in a side cup of salad dressing every 3–4 mouthfuls of salad and you'll enjoy the taste without the extra calories.

12. **Teflon coated pans** and the new **edible spray-on coatings** which are made of vegetable oil will help reduce the amount of caloric fat that you consume. Although **margarine** is lower in saturated fats than butter, it is still 100% fat and has almost as many calories as butter.

13. **Alcohol:** Alcohol is one of the most serious

hazards in any program, whether it is dining out or at home. The additional calories which are consumed in the American diet from alcohol have a tendency to cause and maintain overweight problems. Alcohol has more calories (7 calories per gram) than most foods on a weight basis. Try to substitute club soda with a twist of lemon or mineral water for drinks. When you do have to have a drink, drink a small amount of white wine or a light beer.

WHY DO WE GET FOOD CRAVINGS?

Food cravings may have a **physiological** as well as an **emotional** component, according to many researchers. Those eating binges or cravings for ice cream, pizza, and hoagies may not necessarily begin in the stomach.

CARBOHYDRATE CRAVINGS for sweets, cakes, pretzels, potato chips and crackers may be caused by **low blood sugar.** This condition can occur when you have not eaten for several hours or because of emotional frustration and has been noted to be present prior to the menstrual period because of hormonal fluctuations. Small frequent **high protein meals** can cut or reduce this carbohydrate craving.

SALT CRAVINGS such as pickles, potato chips, and olives can result from a **salt depletion** caused by excessive perspiration, or a **stress condition** which results in an alteration of the adrenal glands. Salt cravings can be reduced by substituting lemon juice and herbs and adding fresh fruit (orange, grapefruit, banana, cantaloupe, tomatoes or strawberries) to the diet which has a **high vitamin C content** and is thought to reduce the craving for salt.

CAFFEINE is present in coffee, tea, cola drinks, cocoa and chocolate (theobromine—a caffeine-type substance). Many people are actually **addicted** both physiologically and metabolically to caffeine and will suffer emotional **withdrawal symptoms** which include headache, fatigue, nausea, irritability and even a craving for sugar. To reduce this addiction you have to gradually reduce the caffeine in your diet by substituting **non-caffeine drinks** such as decaffeinated coffee, herbal teas, clear diet sodas other than colas, and mineral water or club soda.

THOSE SNEAKY, HIDDEN FATS KEEP GETTING IN OUR FOOD

The typical **American diet** is considerably higher in fat content than nearly any other country in the world. There is little doubt that this increased fat intake in our diet is responsible for such diseases as heart disease, obesity, cancers of the colon, breast and prostate. **Fat** is the most concentrated source of calories since a gram of dietary fat supplies your body with **9 calories.** This compares to only 4 calories per gram of protein or carbohydrate. Alcohol has 7 calories per gram, even less than fat, but more than carbohydrate or protein. Since fat has this concentrated source of calories, it is the **most fattening type of food** that we consume and it stands to reason that cutting down on the fat intake is one of the best ways to cut down on the total amount of calories and maintain normal body weight.

Fat accounted for approximately 30% of our calories in the early 1900's, whereas today the fat content of our diet has more than 40% of our calories coming from fat.

In order to meet the basic nutritional requirements, we need only eat one tablespoon of **polyunsaturated oil** each day, which supplies the essential fatty acid called **linoleic acid.** This essential fatty acid helps you absorb fat-soluble vitamins. Americans, however, eat 6 to 8 times this amount of fat, and fat can be considered to be the major source of nutritionally empty calories for most Americans.

Americans have become more conscious of fat consumption in the past 10 years; however, only about a **third** of the fat we eat is **visible** fat, such as hard fat on meat, fats and oils used in cooking, and oil-based salad dressings. Most of the fat in our diet, unfortunately, is **hidden fat** and not as readily noticeable as the marbled fat on meat.

Hidden fat, unfortunately, is a major part of hard cheeses, cream cheese, deep-fried foods, creamed soups, ice cream, chocolate, nuts and seeds. Hidden fat is also a major ingredient of processed, prepared foods such as baked goods (pies, cakes and cookies), processed meats (bologna, hot dogs, etc.), coffee creamers, whipped toppings, snack foods and instant meals.

Many health food products which are purchased as substitutes for saturated fats have in themselves high fat content. Nuts and seeds, sesame paste, granola, quiches and avocados may contain more than half the calories as fat calories.

REDUCING FAT IN YOUR DIET

When shopping in the market it is often difficult to tell how much fat is contained in the processed foods. Always check the label for the ingredients and remember that the **ingredients** are listed in **order of their weight.** Therefore, if fat is listed as one of the first two ingredients, then the product is likely to be high in fat, especially if it precedes the flour content in such items as cakes and pies.

FATS

Whipped margarine and butter contain less fat per

serving than regular margarine or butter because air or water replaces some of the fat in these products. A tablespoon of mayonnaise or oil may have as many fat calories as a teaspoon of hard fat; however, the softer more liquid fats are less saturated.

DAIRY PRODUCTS

Low fat 1% milk or skim milk is preferable to any other milk product. Low fat yogurt, cottage cheese and ricotta cheese are preferable to other dairy products. Parmesan and mozzarella cheese made from skimmed milk have less fat than hard cheeses. Sour cream and sweet cream both are high in fat content and should be avoided. Use skimmed milk if you are preparing puddings or custards from a packaged mix.

Ice milk and frozen yogurt have less fat than ice cream and milkshakes. Soft ice cream, such as frozen custard, may contain as much fat as the hard varieties. Buttermilk contains little or no butter fat and can be used in baked goods to add taste and richness.

SALADS

Salads are fine for the low fat diet provided they are made without dressings—use herbs and spices. Occasionally adding lemon juice with the spices will be satisfactory. There are also low calorie salad dressings which can be used; however, they too have a considerable fat content.

SOUPS

Clear consomme broth and clear soup made with noodles, rice or vegetables are preferable to creamed soups or heavy stock soups.

MEATS

Heavily marbled prime cuts of meats and processed meats are the highest in fat content. Sirloin tip, london broil and flank steak are leaner than the heavily marbled beef. Veal and leg of lamb are also lean. Always buy lean hamburger.

Never fry meats, always broil or grill. Avoid gravies or cream sauces. Make gravy at home after skimming off the fat.

FISH

Tuna and salmon, surprisingly, are among the fattier fishes. Sardines in oil and many forms of smoked fish are also high in fat content. Fresh fish, in particular flounder, cod, halibut, perch, haddock, and sole, have considerably less fat. Tuna packed in water has approximately ⅓ the fat content of tuna packed in oil. Shell-fish, surprisingly, although having a high cholesterol content are low in saturated fats; however, they should be used in moderation.

POULTRY

Poultry should also be broiled or grilled, rather than fried. Discard the skin of poultry, preferably before cooking so as to avoid the saturated fats being absorbed into the carcass of the poultry. Do not use creamed sauces or gravies. Always trim off skin before eating any poultry product.

VEGETABLES

Vegetables fortunately are a low source of hidden dietary fat. In many cases they can be substituted for protein because of the protein content of many vegetable products. Dried beans and peas (kidney beans, split peas, lentils and bean curd) are particularly high in fiber content and low in fat and of moderate protein value. All other vegetables and fruits are without saturated fat content and are excellent sources of carbohydrate for the body.

BAKED GOODS

Commercially prepared baked goods contain considerable saturated fat. The one exception to this is angel food cake. Sweetened fig bars, vanilla wafers and gingersnaps have less fat than cookies and cakes made with chocolate or cream fillings.

Biscuits, muffins, croissants and butter rolls are high in fat content. English muffins, French or Italian breads are lower in fat content. Breadsticks, matzos and crisps are low fat substitutes for most crackers which are high in fat content. Popcorn is one of the most suitable of the low fat, low calorie snack foods.

NOW YOU'RE COOKING WITH STEAM!

While all cooking methods decrease nutrients to some degree, the loss of vitamins, minerals, proteins, and nutritional value is considerably less with steam cooking compared to boiling. The **water soluble vitamins** that are retained when cooking with steam are significant. Broccoli retains only 33% of its vitamin C when boiled compared to 79% retained with steam cooking. Asparagus retains 43% vitamin C compared to 78% when steamed; beans retain 43% with boiling compared to 75% with steam cooking.

When nutrients are lost during boiling, so is the **color** and **flavor** of most foods. Steam cooking preserves the flavor whereas boiling usually disperses the flavor into the cooking water along with the nutrients.

Steam cooking is considerably **faster** than other methods of cooking and, in turn, saves considerable energy. The new type electric steamer, which allows stacking, makes it possible to cook several different foods at one time with a considerable saving of both time and energy. The stainless steel fold-out steamer and the bamboo steamer are both inexpensive and easy to use.

Fish, poultry and vegetables are excellent dishes to prepare with steam cooking. There are many excellent books and manuals on cooking with steam and they can offer you a variety of suggestions and dishes for this excellent, healthful type of food preparation.

POPCORN: THE HIGH FIBER, LOW CHOLESTEROL, LOW CALORIE SNACK

Without the added salt, oil and butter, popcorn is probably one of the best diet snacks available. It is **low in calories and cholesterol** and **high in fiber.** It consequently fills you up without adding extra calories and provides the necessary fiber for proper intestinal function. One cup of popcorn contains only 25 calories. This is why I have included popcorn as your mid-evening snack.

The **electric hot-air popper** is, by far, the most efficient way to prepare popcorn. Since it uses no oil, there are no added fats and there is no cleanup necessary. These hot-air poppers can produce great quantities of popcorn in a relatively short period of time. This electric appliance is a must for your low cholesterol, high fiber walking diet.

There are a number of **combinations** that can be used with popcorn to add flavor and variety to this low calorie snack:

1. Popcorn can be eaten as a breakfast cereal with fruit, skim milk and a teaspoon of wheat germ.
2. Popcorn croutons: Popcorn can be utilized in salads and soups in place of croutons.
3. Popcorn and peanuts: Popcorn and peanuts (dry, unsalted roasted peanuts) can be an excellent evening snack with a glass of diet soda.
4. Popcorn, peanuts and raisins: Same as above.

5. Apple and popcorn: Slices of apple mixed with popcorn can be an ideal snack.
6. Cooking with popcorn: Apple popcorn crisp, chili popcorn, parmesan popcorn, garlic popcorn, peanut butter popcorn balls, raisin or cinnamon popcorn, nut popcorn balls.

Many of these recipes for cooking with popcorn can be found in any of your high fiber diet cookbooks, and should be used only after you've reached your ideal weight.

WHY YOU REALLY NEVER LOSE WEIGHT!

Remember, no one loses weight in a straight line. When you are on a diet, you initially lose weight, and then your weight loss levels off. This occurs even though you are eating exactly the same amount as you were when you lost the weight. This leveling off period or **plateau** is the single most hazardous part of any diet program.

The reason is that once this plateau is reached, you begin to become discouraged and you'll say, "I'm still on the same diet but I haven't lost a pound in over a week." Discouragement leads to frustration and next you'll say, "the heck with the diet, I may as well enjoy myself and eat something I really like since I haven't lost weight anyway." At this point 90% of all diets are doomed to failure since the weight loss pattern now reverses itself and becomes a **weight gain pattern.**

If you can stick out this plateau period, which incidentally is **always temporary,** you'll be surprised to see that the weight loss begins to pick up speed again. It may take a week or two at the most, but if you are patient, you will again start to lose those unwanted pounds.

No one has ever satisfactorily explained this plateau period; however, physiologists believe that it is probably due to a **temporary re-adjustment of the body's metabolism** in response to the initial weight loss. No matter what the reason is, however, you will always break through the plateau period providing you don't become discouraged or frustrated. Weight loss will again resume its downward progress toward your ideal weight goal.

This plateau period is one of the main reasons that I insist that my patients do not weigh themselves daily; in fact, **weighing yourself every day is hazardous to your diet.** Psychiatrists have found that people who weigh themselves daily never lose weight. The reason for this is two-fold. **First,** when you weigh yourself daily and see that you are losing weight, you become happy and elated, and subconsciously you will eat to celebrate. **Secondly,** if you see that you are not losing weight as fast as you "think" you should, you become depressed and anxious, and sometime during that day you will subconsciously eat because of frustration.

So the rule of thumb is: **the more you weigh yourself, the more you eat!** Believe me, it is true. I've seen my patients go through this frustrating daily weighing process thousands of times. No one on a diet should weigh themselves more than once a week and then you will get a true measure of the effectiveness of your diet. **Wednesday** is the best day to weigh yourself each week. Monday and Friday are the worst days for weighing in, since they precede and follow the weekend and lead to frustration-type eating binges. It took a long time to gain all that weight; you can't take it off overnight. Be patient!

6

FEARLESS FIBER: SECRET AGENT

HOW CAN I LIVE LONGER?

In Chapters 3 and 4 you have seen how the **DR.'S F*A*S*T* 3-DAY DIETWALK®** can help you lose weight and stay thin forever. Now we will discuss how this diet program will keep you healthy and help you to live longer (Chapters 6, 7 and 8). Yes, I actually said "live longer."

Medical research has consistently provided studies that show that a high fiber/low cholesterol diet is good for you. There is no longer any doubt about the validity of these reports. In fact, a **high fiber/low cholesterol walking diet** is the only known type of program that we can utilize to add disease-free years to our lives. We can't change our genetic structure; however, we certainly can modify it to improve our odds of survival.

In this chapter (Chapter 6) you will see how **Fearless Fiber** not only slims you down, but prevents at least a dozen diet-related diseases. In Chapter 7 we will show you how **Cholesterol Control** can help you stay thin and trim outside, while keeping your arteries clean as a whistle inside. And in Chapter 8, you will see how avoiding the **Seven Deadly S's** will add years to your life.

WEIGHT REDUCTION BY INCREASING FIBER IN THE DIET

Dietary fiber is the part of plants that is resistant to the breakdown of enzymes in our digestive tract. Many physicians believe that dietary fiber is an extremely important part of our diet and are advising their patients to increase the amount of fiber in their diet by eating more fruits, vegetables and whole grain cereals and breads.

Epidemiologic studies have shown that the western diet has become progressively **fiber deficient** over the past half-century, whereas the diet in under-developed countries is extremely high in fiber. This fact stems from the progressive elimination of fiber (the unabsorbable portion of the plant food) in western diet as a result of the **milling of flour** which removes the outer layer or covering (bran) of the wheat kernel. Bran is one of the most concentrated sources of food fiber.

High-fiber diets have been reported by a major medical university to be **excellent weight reduction diets.** Not only have these diets been effective in treating obese diabetic patients, but they have had marked effects on obese non-diabetics also. The following simplified high-fiber diet has been recommended for weight reduction:

1. Whole grain products (bran and whole grain cereals, and brown long grain rice)
2. Whole grain bread (stone ground or whole wheat)
3. Garden vegetables (carrots, celery, cabbage, green beans, lettuce, onions, corn, peas, tomatoes, potatoes)

4. Fruits (apples, oranges, pears, bananas, strawberries, blueberries, plums, peaches and cher-
   ries)
5. Miller's bran: Miller's bran is a dry wheat
   powder which is a convenient high dietary fiber. Each level teaspoon of miller's bran contains 2 grams of dietary fiber. Miller's bran may
   be sprinkled on cereal or other foods, or it may
   be mixed in with orange or tomato juice to
   improve its taste.

A high-fiber diet is essentially a normal diet which
has been changed to minimize or decrease the intake of
refined foods. This encourages the consumption of
fresh fruits, vegetables, whole grain cereals and
breads. When the fiber is eaten from a variety of food
sources, it produces its most beneficial effect, especially when it is eaten with each meal of the day.

Dietary fiber takes longer to chew and eat with the
subsequent development of more saliva and a larger
bulk swallowed with each mouthful. The larger bulk
helps to fill the stomach and causes a decrease in
hunger before more calories are consumed. High fiber
diets help to provide bulk without energy, and may
reduce the amount of energy absorbed from the food
that is eaten. These high fiber diets are often referred to
as having a low-energy density and appear to prevent
excessive caloric (energy) intake. Countries that consume high fiber diets rarely have obesity problems.

FIBER FACTS

What is fiber? In the first half of the 19th century the
term **crude fiber** was the generally accepted term used
in the food tables. This measurement, however, was not
for human purposes. The definition of crude fiber was
described as the plant food remaining after the food

had been boiled first in acid and then in alkali. Crude fiber includes only a few of the actual fiber components of plants; however, it was the description used on most food packages until recently.

Dietary fiber is a newer measurement and refers to all fiber components of plants including crude fiber. It is therefore a more accurate measurement of the fiber content of foods. The dietary fiber content consequently has a higher numerical reading than grams of crude fiber. Fiber, commonly known as **bulk** or **roughage**, is the part of plant foods that can not be digested completely, so that it passes through the digestive tract intact. Therefore, dietary fiber is the fiber content of food which is resistant to the human digestive enzymes.

The function of fiber: The most important function of dietary fiber is to **bind water** in the intestine in the form of a gel. This gel prevents its over-absorption from the large intestine and insures that the stool content of the large bowel is both bulky and soft and consequently its passage through the intestine is not delayed. Another important function of fiber is its effect on the metabolism, absorption, and reabsorption of **bile acids and cholesterol**. Dietary fiber actually binds or attaches to both cholesterol and bile acid and consequently decreases their absorption from the bowel. It is now recognized that there are a number of diseases and disorders which are, at least in part, caused by a lack of dietary fiber (Burkitt, P.D., Trowell, H.C., eds. Refined Carbohydrate Foods and Disease, New York (London): Academic Press, 1975). These diet-related diseases can be classified as follows:

1. **Gastrointestinal disorders:** constipation, diverticulosis, appendicitis, hiatal hernia, hemorrhoids, cancer of the colon.

2. **Metabolic disorders:** Obesity, diabetes, gallstones.
3. **Cardiovascular disorders:** atherosclerosis (coronary artery disease) and varicose veins.

A recent study has shown that these diseases are now becoming prevalent in non-European communities which have introduced western dietary customs. There is almost an inverse relationship between the amount of fiber consumed and the prevalence of these various diseases in different countries. The higher the intake of dietary fiber, the lower the incidence of the above named disorders.

The latest medical report on high fiber foods indicates that there may possibly be a *cancer-protecting substance* actually contained in some dark green and yellow vegetables and fruits. The substance known as **beta-carotene** (a nutrient that the body converts into vitamin A) is found in high concentration in spinach, carrots, broccoli, Brussels sprouts, cauliflower, winter squash, cabbage, oranges, grapefruit, apricots and peaches. These high fiber foods also contain large amounts of vitamin C. Both vitamins may possibly be protective against cancer of the lung, esophagus, stomach, large bowel and skin in some patients.

DIET DIFFERENCES AROUND THE WORLD

Many epidemiologic studies show that the following **5 BASIC DIETARY CHANGES** distinguish our modern western diet from developing countries:

1. **An increased consumption of salt.** Most western countries consume 10 to 12 grams of salt daily, as opposed to undeveloped nations which consume no more than 1 gram daily.

2. **An increased consumption of fat.** Western countries consume approximately 3 times the amount of fat calories as compared to poorer, under-developed nations.

3. **An increased consumption of refined sugar**, which provides almost half the total carbohydrate calories in the western diet.

4. **A decreased consumption of complex carbohydrates.** Western countries consume not more than 20% complex carbohydrate calories whereas third world developing countries consume more than 70% of their total calories in carbohydrates.

5. **A decreased consumption of fiber** in western diets is one of the most important of these 5 factors which has greatly increased the tendency toward the development of the above mentioned diseases. This decreased intake in fiber has been due in part to the invention of freezing foods and canning. Also, fiber has been deliberately removed in the milling process since it was originally thought to be unimportant and non-nutritious.

DISEASES AND DISORDERS RESULTING FROM LACK OF FIBER

1. **CONSTIPATION:** Constipation results from the delayed passage of stool material which is entirely due to the excess absorption of water from the large bowel. This in turn causes a dry, hard stool which has a delayed passage through the intestinal tract. By preventing **excess absorption of water from the bowel**, dietary fiber increases the passage of a bulky soft stool with a more rapid transit through the intestinal tract. By world standards, Americans are almost universally constipated.

2. **DIVERTICULAR DISEASE OF THE COLON:** Diverticular disease or diverticulosis of the colon is

thought to be caused by an **increased pressure inside the colon**, which results from the muscular effort that is necessary to move the stool along the colon. Abnormally high pressures caused by the lack of dietary fiber and constipation forces small pouches in the lining wall of the large intestine. These are referred to as diverticula or small pockets in the muscular wall of the large intestine.

3. **APPENDICITIS:** While only in the hypothetical stage at this point, many investigators feel that acute appendicitis is a result of a diet low in dietary fiber. This results from **excessive muscle contraction** in the appendix wall and a **blockage** in the appendix by hard, fecal material, both of which result from inadequate dietary fiber.

4. **HIATAL HERNIA:** Hiatal hernia is defined as an upper protrusion of the top of the stomach through the diaphragm into the upper chest cavity. Constipation not only increases the pressure within the bowel itself but also within the abdomen during the straining at stool. These **increased pressures** are believed to force the junction of the esophagus and stomach upward into the chest cavity.

5. **CANCER OF THE COLON:** Some people seem to have an excessive amount of **bile acids** in the colon, on which bacteria may act to produce cancer producing agents, in particular **nitrates** or **nitrosamines**. The current theory is that an increased amount of dietary fiber will produce a large fecal volume, which will dilute these carcinogens and make their transit more rapid through the bowel, thus giving them less time to adhere or stick to the bowel wall and exert their cancer producing qualities.

6. **HEMORRHOIDS:** Hemorrhoids are thought to be caused by the **increased intra-abdominal pressure** transmitted from the abdominal veins during straining at stool to the anal veins. Constipation resulting from a

lack of dietary fiber also produces a **shearing stress** when passing hard stools, causing the attachments of the anal veins to become stretched. One out of every two Americans over the age of 50 is plagued by rectal hemorrhoids. In England, patients with hemorrhoids are almost never referred to surgeons, but are routinely treated with high fiber diets.

7. **GALLSTONES:** Gallstones occasionally result from bile which is overloaded with a **crystalloid type of cholesterol**. There is evidence that dietary fiber reduces the cholesterol and increases the more beneficial components of the bile, thus reducing the tendency toward stone formation.

8. **DIABETES:** Low-carbohydrate diets are being replaced by diets higher in carbohydrates, particularly the **complex starches or carbohydrates**. Refined sugars are almost totally eliminated from this type of diet. Since this diet is higher in fiber, the intestinal content becomes more gelatinous (thicker) and subsequently slows the absorption of energy (and sugar) from the intestinal tract. This has a protective effect against the development of either high or low blood sugar levels after eating, since slow absorption makes for a more even distribution of sugar in the blood. Diabetes is rarely found in populations that consume high levels of dietary fiber.

9. **OBESITY:** High fiber foods such as fruits, vegetables, nuts and bran cereals generally require a longer time to eat since they require more **chewing** and tend to be **bulky**. This may help to create a feeling of fullness. With foods that are low in dietary fiber, more food is ingested before a sense of fullness has been attained. This food is usually eaten more rapidly, requires less chewing, is not bulky in character, and, therefore, enters the stomach more rapidly. Since it takes time for nerve impulses to reach the appetite control center, the feeling of hunger is not shut off until

excessive amounts of low dietary fiber foods are eaten, and obesity is almost certain to result.

10. **VARICOSE VEINS:** There is strong evidence to indicate that straining at stool caused by lack of dietary fiber increases the intra-abdominal pressure and these pressures are directly transmitted to the veins draining the leg. Repeated high pressures caused by straining enlarges these veins, stretching their **small valves**, which normally prevent the leakage of blood backwards in the veins. Since it is these valves which assist the upward flow of blood, their loss of function combined with gravity raises the pressure in the veins of the legs and results in varicose veins. Approximately 35% of pregnant American women develop varicose veins, compared to less than 5% of pregnant women in countries consuming high fiber diets.

11. **CORONARY HEART DISEASE:** Dietary fiber binds with bile acids and cholesterol in the intestinal tract and subsequently reduces their absorption from the bowel into the blood stream. This may help to explain why in under-developed countries with a high proportion of dietary fiber there is a low prevalence of coronary heart disease. On a high fiber diet, studies show that **blood fats** were significantly reduced (cholesterol was reduced 25% and triglycerides 15%).

12. **BREAST DISEASE:** Recent studies have indicated that there may be a relationship between constipation and breast disease. This is based on the fact that either substances which are **carcinogenic** or female **hormones** may enter the blood stream from the colon and reach the breast tissue. These substances may then have a stimulating effect by producing either benign cystic breast disease and possibly cancer of the breast tissue. Dietary fiber may possibly play an indirect role in the prevention of these disorders.

SIDE EFFECTS OF HIGH FIBER DIETS

Up to this point, we have talked about the many benefits and advantages of the high fiber diet. We must now
turn to possible side effects of high fiber diets. The
following side effects have been reported in the medical literature and, while not serious, deserve mention-
ing:

1. The most common side effect of the high fiber
diet is marked **flatulence**. This especially manifests itself by a sensation of bloating, gas, and occasionally
abdominal pain and diarrhea. These symptoms can be
decreased or minimized if you drink plenty of liquids
during the day and gradually increase the dietary fiber
in divided doses over a period of three to four weeks,
so that the bowel can adjust to this new component.

2. There have been studies using large doses of
purified fiber, indicating that there is a loss of some
trace minerals, notably zinc, calcium, copper, iron, and
magnesium, which appear to be bound by fiber and
subsequently eliminated in the feces (American Journal of Clinical Nutrition, 31:S21, 1978; 32: 1893, 1979).
It appears unlikely that a mineral deficiency will develop in people who have a balanced diet and consume
moderate amounts of dietary fiber not exceeding 20–25
grams daily.

3. Patients who have **stomach or intestinal problems** should not be given a high fiber diet because of
the possible risk of irritation of the intestinal wall and
the remote possibility of intestinal obstruction. Check
with your physician first.

4. **Diabetic** patients should be cautioned that
when they are put on a high fiber diet, they may need
less insulin or oral diabetic agents (Annals of Internal

Medicine, 88: 482, 1978). They should first check with their physician before starting a high fiber diet.

Diets that contain no more than **20 grams** of dietary fiber pose little problems to health. There have been no significant reported side effects with diets containing fiber content of 20 grams or less. Remember, the average American diet contains no more than 7–8 grams of dietary fiber, so you should start slowly and gradually increase the amount of fiber in your diet to minimize any possible side effects. It is important to check with your own physician before starting any diet program.

If you can't get enough fiber (15–20 grams) in your food on any particular day because of restaurant dining, business trips, vacations, etc., you can still get your daily fiber quota by eating either of the following:

1. 1–2 tbsp. Miller's bran in juice, milk, water or sprinkled on any food (each tbsp. supplies **6** gms. dietary fiber).
2. 1–2 FIBERMED™ Wafers made by The Purdue Frederick Co.® (each wafer supplies **5** gms. dietary fiber).

HIGH FIBER FOODS

FRUIT GROUP: Each serving of the below named fruits has approximately 2 grams of fiber.

apple	1 pear
banana	1 medium peach
½ cup of strawberries	2 small plums
1 small orange	10 large cherries

BREAD GROUP: Each serving has approximately 2 grams of fiber.

whole wheat bread	bran muffin
wheat bread (cracked)	stone ground bread

CEREAL GROUP: Each serving has approximately 2 grams of fiber.

shredded wheat—½ biscuit	oatmeal 3 tbsps.
puffed wheat—1⅓ cups	wheat bran—1 tsp.
corn flakes—⅔ cup	grape nuts—3 tbsps.

Cereals highest in fiber are 40% Bran, All Bran, GrapeNuts, Shredded Wheat, Whole Wheat Flakes, Raisin Bran.

VEGETABLES GROUP: Each serving has approximately 2 grams of fiber.

celery—1 cup	2 cups of lettuce
1 corn on the cob—2 inches	½ cup green beans
2 tbsps. baked beans	1 medium potato
1 medium raw tomato	4 Brussels sprouts
½ stalk of broccoli	⅓ cup carrots

The following vegetables are highest in fiber: artichokes, green beans, cabbage, cauliflower, Brussels sprouts, dried peas and beans, lima beans, and peas.

MISCELLANEOUS GROUP: Each serving has approximately 1 gram of fiber.

2½ tsps. of peanut butter	10 peanuts
5 tbsps. of strawberry jam	1 large pickle

The following miscellaneous items also have higher than average fiber content: popcorn, chunky peanut butter, relishes.

For additional information on fiber see **APPENDIX** for the **FIBER AND CALORIE COUNTER.**

7

CRIMINAL CHOLESTEROL: HEART ATTACKER

FAT PEOPLE DIE YOUNG

In a study just released by the National Heart, Lung, and Blood Institute in Bethesda, MD, **obesity** has now been listed as a **major independent risk factor** for **heart disease.** What's so new about that? Everyone knows that being overweight contributes to heart disease. That's just it; up until now obesity was just a contributing factor in heart disease because of its relationship with high blood pressure and high cholesterol. Now it has gained its own independent rating as causing heart disease all by itself. This study, consisting of **5,000 men and women** was followed for **26 years.** According to Dr. Helen B. Hubert, the risk of developing heart disease was more pronounced in people who gained most of their excess weight after the **age of 25.**

In this study **obesity ranked 3rd in men and 4th in women** in predicting **coronary heart disease.** The other risk factors in heart disease were high blood pressure, serum cholesterol, cigarette smoking, age, diabetes and electrocardiogram abnormalities. Only high blood pressure, cholesterol and age were ranked ahead of obesity with cigarette smoking a close 4th in predicting heart disease. One important point made in this extensive study was: losing a moderate amount of weight **lessened the risk of developing heart disease.**

AMERICAN HEART ASSOCIATION REPORT 1982 (Heart Facts 1982)

According to the American Heart Association, more than 41 million Americans have one or more forms of heart or blood vessel disease.

Heart attacks claimed 550,000 lives in 1979, 56% of all deaths from cardiovascular disease. The Heart Association estimated that as many as 1 million Americans will have a heart attack this year and more than one-third of them will die.

Stroke was listed as the second leading cause of death in cardiovascular disease which claimed 170,000 lives in 1979. They estimated that 1.8 million Americans are survivors of stroke.

High blood pressure: one in every four adults or 35 million Americans suffer from high blood pressure. In 1979 over 30 thousand people died from the complications of high blood pressure.

Cardiovascular disease accounts for more than 45% of all deaths which occur in the United States yearly, and in most cases is caused by atherosclerosis. Since obesity is often associated with elevated blood cholesterol levels, it is thought to be indirectly responsible for the development of atherosclerosis (fat deposits in arteries). Recent studies also indicate that obesity also increases the risk of developing hypertension. In many mild cases of high blood pressure, weight loss alone can serve as an effective treatment. The following charts—FACTS ABOUT FAT—will illustrate what happens inside your body as fat accumulates (Figs. 1 & 2).

FACTS ABOUT FAT
Figure 1

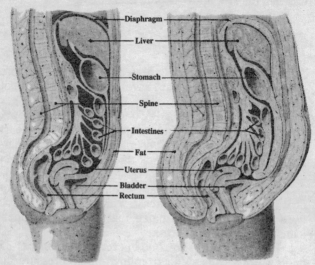

NORMAL   **OVERWEIGHT**

© Romaine Pierson Pubs., Inc. Courtesy of *Medical Times*

If you have a weight problem—controlled or uncontrolled—you are not alone. There are about 15 million Americans who are at least 20% overweight, and that's borderline obesity. The more your weight goes up, the more problems you'll encounter in maintaining health and achieving longevity. "The longer the waistline, the shorter the lifeline" is an all too familiar adage. But sadly, it doesn't really sink in for many people until the insidious growth of girth creates a crisis. This chart shows what happens *inside* your body as you progress from being slightly overweight to being obese. We're not stressing the cosmetic disabilities caused by excess weight—or the psychological problems. We are presenting the gut problem.

Shortness of breath may be a first sign of pulmonary distress and heart strain caused by overweight. The chart shows you how and why obesity increases the heart's workload and contributes to pre-

FACTS ABOUT FAT
Figure 2

NORMAL AMOUNT OF FAT

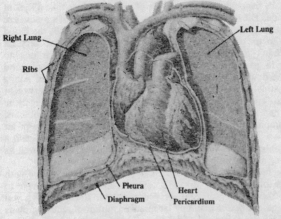

EXCESS AMOUNT OF FAT

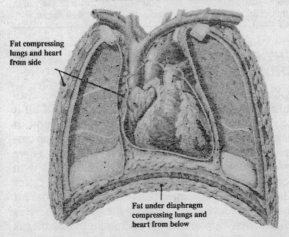

mature death: fat enlarges the capillary bed (tiny connective blood vessels in an area or organ of your body) which increases the amount of tissue to be nourished by the blood and through which the blood must be pumped by your heart.

In addition, the fat accumulated has to go someplace. You can see what's happening on the outside of you—now let's take a look at the inside. Fat infiltrates the liver and other organs. It's a squeeze process, an invasion. Fat compresses the heart, decreases the blood supply to the intestines, etc. (See figures above.) Some very fat people can't sit, because if they do, there's no space for their lungs to operate in, as the fat invades the chest. These people have to stand up or lie down all the time. They have disabled themselves. Along with all this, extra heavy people—and even moderately overweight persons—are putting an extra burden on their backs and legs (the weight bearing joints), which causes or increases arthritic problems.

Complications following surgery occur more frequently in fat people vs. thin. Wounds don't heal as well or as fast. And again a breathing problem—heavyweights can't take anesthesia as well as people of normal weight.

The final point to remember is that weight will always be with you—as long as you're alive. To control your weight, you have to control the number of calories you eat. Your doctor knows you inside and out better than any far-removed author of reducing plans that please the palate. Your doctor will prescribe a highly individualized diet—just for you—to help you beat the battle of the bulge, which this chart should show you goes on inside as well as out.

WEIGHT CONTROL BY CONTROLLING INTAKE OF CHOLESTEROL

Controlling our weight by reducing the amount of cholesterol in our diet has a twofold benefit. First of all it will help control and maintain our weight. Second, it will have a beneficial effect on the prevention of cardiovascular and cerebral-vascular disease, since, as we have seen, these illnesses have been associated with high levels of blood cholesterol.

The typical **American diet** has a higher fat content than nearly any other country in the world. There is little doubt that this increased fat intake in our diet is responsible for the development of **obesity,** as well as many other disorders. **Fat** is the most concentrated source of calories since a gram of dietary fat supplies your body with **9 calories.** This compared to only 4 calories per gram of protein or carbohydrate. Since fat has this concentrated source of calories, it is the **most fattening** type of food that we consume and it stands to reason that cutting down on the fat intake is one of the best ways to cut down on the total amount of calories and maintain normal body weight.

All foods that are of **plant origin** do not contain cholesterol. These include fruits, vegetables, grains, cereals, nuts, and vegetable oils (coconut and palm oil are the only exceptions). In choosing vegetable oils, make sure that you choose liquid or unsaturated vegetable oils, rather than solid or hydrogenated vegetable oil products, since these liquid oils have a beneficial effect in helping to lower blood cholesterol.

WHAT IS CHOLESTEROL?

Cholesterol is a **fat-like substance** normally found in all living tissue and is an essential chemical for health. It is found in every cell and fluid in the body. Although it resembles fat in many ways, it has a completely different chemical structure called *steroid lipids*. Cholesterol also differs from fat in that it is not used by the body as food for the production of energy.

Cholesterol is extremely important, however, in the **metabolism of fat** and the production of **hormones** in the body. It is equally important in the formation of **bile salts** which aid in our digestion. **Cholesterol** also forms an important structural component of **membranes** (walls) of all the body's cells.

Since the body requires a certain amount of cholesterol all the time, it is manufactured naturally in our bodies, primarily in the liver. So, what's the problem? It looks as if cholesterol is pretty good for our health. Well it is, providing there's not too much of it. Unfortunately, we also get cholesterol into our bodies in the food we eat and that is where the problem begins.

Medical research has shown that when we take in **too much cholesterol** in our diets, the amount of cholesterol in our blood begins to rise. Once there is an excessive amount of cholesterol circulating in our blood stream, it starts to build up in the walls of the arteries. These yellow-rubbery deposits of cholesterol called **plaques** narrow the passageway of the artery (hardening of the arteries). This condition often leads to **heart attacks** and **strokes** since not enough blood can get through these narrowed blood vessels.

WHAT IS SATURATED FAT?

It is present in all products of **animal origin**—meat, fish, fowl, eggs, butter, milk, cream and cheese. Saturated fats are also found in **vegetable products** which are usually solid or semi-solid at room temperature. They include **shortenings** and **table spreads** which have been changed from liquid fats (usually cottonseed and soybean oils) into solids by a process called **hydrogenation.** This process makes the products more suitable for table use and prevents them from becoming rancid. However, this process converts polyunsaturated fats into **saturated fats.**

Other saturated fats in the vegetable kingdom include **cocoa butter, palm oil** and **coconut oil.** Most people are unaware of the fact that they consume considerable amounts of coconut and palm oil. They are used commercially in a wide variety of processed foods, baked goods and deep-fat fried products.

Saturated fats are dangerous because they can increase the amount of **cholesterol** in the blood. These fats can raise the level of blood cholesterol as much as, if not more than, the actual consumption of dietary cholesterol products.

There are four factors that can help to **lower your blood cholesterol** which we will be discussing in this chapter:

1. Decrease the amount of **dietary cholesterol** that you eat.
2. Decrease the amount of **saturated fat** in your diet.
3. Increase the amount of **polyunsaturated fats** in your diet.
4. Continue **THE DOCTOR'S F*A*S*T* 3-DAY DIETWALK®.**

WHAT ARE UNSATURATED FATS?

1. **Monosaturated fats** (neutral fats) have essentially **no effect on your blood cholesterol level.** They are usually liquid at room temperature and tend to harden or cloud when refrigerated. They are the primary fats found in **olive oil, peanut oil** and most **nuts.** They are also present in small amounts in meats, dairy products and some vegetables.
2. **Polyunsaturated fats** (essential fatty acids) are always of **vegetable origin** and are **liquid oils. Safflower oil** is the highest in polyunsaturates of all oils. Sunflower oil is second, followed by corn oil, sesame seed oil, soybean oil, cottonseed oil, walnut oil and linseed oil.

Polyunsaturated fats help to **lower the blood cholesterol level** by assisting the body to eliminate excessive amounts of newly manufactured cholesterol. Don't just add polyunsaturated fats to your diet. It is essential that you substitute polyunsaturated fats for saturated fats to maximize their cholesterol-lowering effect.

It is interesting to note that we can manufacture saturated fat and most monosaturated fats in our bodies. However, polyunsaturated fats must be obtained from the diet and are, therefore, called **essential fatty acids.**

WHAT ARE LIPIDS?

The term lipids is used to include **all fats** and **fat-like substances** (e.g., cholesterol). These lipids will not dissolve in water and are called **fat-soluble** substances. How do they get absorbed into the blood stream, since the blood is a water-soluble solution? These lipids (fats and cholesterol) hook up with certain proteins so that they can dissolve in water (in this case, the blood) and are now called **LIPOPROTEINS.** The protein acts as the submarine, transporting its passenger, Mr. Fat or Mr. Cholesterol, through the blood stream.

There are several types of lipo-protein combinations present in our bodies: however, for our purposes we will discuss two of the most important ones.

1. The **BAD-CHOLESTEROL-SUBMARINE** (LDL—low density lipo-protein combination). This bad submarine (LDL) deposits cholesterol in your arteries when too much cholesterol is taken into the diet or manufactured by the body. You can help here by **eating less cholesterol-rich foods.** The bad submarine will have less cholesterol to carry and therefore won't be able to clog up your arteries with it.

2. The **GOOD-CHOLESTEROL-SUBMARINE** (HDL—high density lipo-protein combination)

is quite a different story. It acts opposite to the bad submarine, by collecting the excess amounts of cholesterol in the blood and taking it to the liver where it is eliminated from the body in the bile juices. Some medical investigators also feel that this good submarine (**HDL**) may be able to take the cholesterol out of the cholesterol deposits (plaques) that have already formed in your arteries in the early stages.

Well, how do we get some of this good **HDL**? It almost sounds too good to be true! As always, there's got to be a catch. First, heredity plays an important part in **HDL** production. Some of us have more than others because of good genes. There's nothing we can do about that. Secondly, diet plays almost no role in affecting **HDL** production—so our low cholesterol diet won't help us here. Smoking, incidentally, has been shown to lower **HDL**—another nail in its coffin.

Fortunately, there is one thing that we can do to raise **HDL** production in our bodies. Medical research has definitely shown that a regular program of a moderate intensity exercise—WALKING—can raise our **HDL** levels. This type of exercise must be continued on a regular basis in order to keep this **HDL** elevated. Short bursts of exercise (high intensity exercise, e.g., jogging) only temporarily raise the **HDL** level and it decreases abruptly after the exercise is stopped. The lifetime walking diet program is the best and only answer to this problem.

LOW CHOLESTEROL DIET STILL ADVISED TO PREVENT CORONARY HEART DISEASE

Since the recent **cholesterol controversy** that was recorded in late 1981, there has been a decrease in interest by many patients and physicians in the relationship of dietary cholesterol and the development of coronary heart disease. Recently, however, the role of cholesterol in the development of heart disease has been definitely established.

There is little doubt that the risk of **coronary heart disease** increases as the level of blood cholesterol rises. Although the increased blood cholesterol may only represent one of the many factors related to the development of coronary artery or heart disease, it is still a significant one.

In **vegetarians** who have blood cholesterol levels of no more than 150 mg. there is essentially no risk of heart disease. Your risk, however, is increased 2 to 3 times when blood levels approach 250 to 300 mg., which incidentally is the range of the blood cholesterol found in the average American.

There have been many studies over the past twenty years which have proven that the **reduction of dietary saturated fat and cholesterol** results in a significant reduction in coronary heart disease. Even reducing the serum cholesterol by 15 to 20% results in a significant decrease in your risk for developing coronary heart disease and other complications of atherosclerosis.

There is also strong evidence that the reduction of saturated fat and cholesterol in the diet may actually **reverse the process of atherosclerosis** (hardening of the arteries). There have been several studies with monkeys where atherosclerotic plaques actually decreased with dietary reduction of saturated fat and cholesterol. There is also strong evidence that this reversal process also may occur in humans by using dietary measures to reduce the blood level of cholesterol. Don't let cholesterol make a monkey out of you!

CHOLESTEROL AND ITS ASSOCIATION WITH HEART DISEASE

1. **Animal studies** show that when laboratory animals are put on a standard, high cholesterol American diet, they develop atherosclerosis or hardening of the coronary arteries. They have considerably less heart disease when they are placed on cholesterol lowering diets and/or medications to lower cholesterol.

2. **The Framingham Heart Study,** which has been in progress since 1948 and has followed over 5,000 people, has repeatedly shown that blood cholesterol level is one of the strongest predictors of a person's risk for developing coronary heart disease. In this study, this is coupled with other risk factors such as blood pressure, smoking, family history, and lack of exercise.

3. In people who have **heart disease** at very young ages or in families where there is a high prevalence of heart disease, cholesterol levels are usually found to be high. Epidemiological studies comparing different nations and cultures show that populations who have a high fat intake have significantly more heart disease than cultures with less fat in their diets. In addition, when certain ethnic groups migrate to a new cultural society, they tend to develop both the cholesterol blood levels and risks of heart disease of their new environments. This suggests that environmental factors such as high cholesterol diets may be more crucial than genetic factors in determining the risk of developing heart disease.

4. The microscopic examination of the **coronary arteries** taken from autopsies shows that cholesterol is always present in the areas where the coronary arteries were blocked. Studies also indicate that this cho-

lesterol found in these areas of blockage has moved into the vessel wall from the blood stream.

There appears to be little doubt from this evidence that the relationship of high levels of **blood cholesterol** to the development of **coronary heart disease** is a significant risk factor. The major factor in reducing the level of cholesterol in the blood is to reduce the amount of **total fat in the diet** (dietary cholesterol and saturated fats). This usually means switching from fatty meats and pork products to leaner meats, fish and poultry. Also, one should reduce the amount of dairy fat in the diet, switching from whole to skim milk and avoiding the use of butter and cream.

A second important factor in determining the level of blood cholesterol is the **type of fat** eaten. Most animal fats are saturated fats, whereas most vegetable oils are **polyunsaturated fats.** Studies have shown that substituting polyunsaturated for saturated fats does result in lowering the blood cholesterol level, even if the total amount of fat in the diet is the same.

And last but not least, is your lifetime **walking** program. Walking not only provides cardiovascular fitness, but as we have seen it also raises the **HDL** (good-cholesterol-submarine) level in our blood. HDL seems to protect our coronary arteries from accumulating too much cholesterol.

THE SEVEN COUNTRIES STUDY

One of the most striking studies on the relationship of **serum cholesterol** to the development of **coronary heart disease** is illustrated in **The Seven Countries Study.**

This study was a collaborative international study of more than **12,000 men, ages 40 to 59 years of age.** Its purpose was to relate the characteristics of these populations to the subsequent development of coronary heart disease. Total communities were involved in the following countries: Greece, Yugoslavia, Italy, Japan, Finland, The Netherlands and the United States.

Dietary differences studied in The Seven Countries Study revealed that people in Japan and the Mediterranean countries consumed a diet containing **10% or less** calories daily from saturated fat, whereas the diet in the United States, Finland and The Netherlands contained **15 to 22% saturated fat.** In the countries that consumed a diet containing 10% or less calories from saturated fat, their dietary consumption of complex carbohydrates and vegetable protein from grains, vegetables, legumes and fruits was significantly higher than in the countries which had a higher intake of saturated fat. The blood cholesterol of people in the **Mediterranean countries and Japan was 200 mg. or less,** whereas in the **United States, Finland and The Netherlands,** whose intake of saturated fats was approximately 20% of calories, the blood cholesterol levels ranged from **230 to 265 mg.**

The **blood cholesterol levels** in the seven countries studied were directly correlated with the incidence of **coronary heart disease. Japan,** which had the lowest incidence of coronary heart disease in this study, had the lowest blood cholesterol level of about 160 mg. **East Finland,** on the other hand, had the highest rate of coronary heart disease and had the highest serum cholesterol level, approximately 260 mg.

The 10 year mortality from coronary heart disease was lowest in **Japan** and the **three Mediterranean countries** (Yugoslavia, Greece and Italy). The highest rates were found in the **United States** and **Finland.**

There can be little doubt from this intensive, exhaustive study that the level of serum cholesterol which is directly related to the intake of **saturated fat and dietary cholesterol** is a prime risk factor in the development of **coronary heart disease.**

DON'T BELIEVE THE NEW INSURANCE WEIGHT CHARTS!

The recently revised insurance weight tables have created considerable controversy among the medical profession, since they were released early in 1983. The revised weights are 5–15 lbs. heavier than the 1959 tables. Most medical authorities, including The American Heart Association, strongly disagree with these recommendations. They are advising their patients to adhere to the 1959 desirable weight limits.

Obesity has now been classified as an independent risk factor in the development of cardiovascular disease. Being over-weight also is a contributing factor in the development of hypertension, diabetes, stroke, kidney disease and heart attacks. Considering these factors, most medical authorities agree that it does not make sense to raise the limits for recommended weights.

CHOLESTEROL CONTENT OF FOODS

MEAT, FISH AND POULTRY HIGH IN CHOLESTEROL

fatty cuts beef, pork, ham, veal and mutton

duck, goose

organ meats (kidney, liver, heart, sweetbread and brain)

luncheon meats and canned meats; sausage

sardines, herring

shell fish (shrimp, lobster, crab, clams, oysters, scallops)

MEAT, FISH AND POULTRY LOW IN CHOLESTEROL

chicken and turkey
without skin
fresh fish (flounder,
cod, bass, sole,
perch, haddock,
halibut, salmon,
trout, tuna, carp,
pike)

tuna and salmon
packed in water or
with oil drained
lean ground meat and
very lean cuts of
beef, pork, ham and
veal

DAIRY PRODUCTS HIGH IN CHOLESTEROL

whole milk
evaporated milk
butter
cheeses
eggs

creams (sour, whipped,
half & half, ice
cream, cheeses made
from whole milk or
cream)
dairy coffee creamers

DAIRY PRODUCTS LOW IN CHOLESTEROL

non-fat or skimmed
milk
low-fat buttermilk
canned evaporated non-
fat milk
margarines high in
polyunsaturates
egg substitutes
(Fleischmann's Egg
Beaters®)

yogurt (low fat)
cocoa
cheeses made from
skimmed milk
egg white

low-fat cheeses

low-fat cottage cheese

BREAD AND CEREALS HIGH IN CHOLESTEROL

commercial muffins
biscuits

rolls and buns
coffee cakes

donuts

mixes containing whole milk, butter and eggs

crackers

white bread

corn bread

BREAD AND CEREALS LOW IN CHOLESTEROL

whole wheat, French, Italian, pumpernickel and rye breads

homemade cookies, muffins and biscuits, if made with margarine or polyunsaturated oil

cereals, hot and cold (whole grain and bran type, served with low-fat milk)

English muffins

bran muffins

matzo, soda crackers, bread sticks

OTHER FOODS LOW IN CHOLESTEROL

most fish except shell fish

pastas, noodles and rice—whole grain types

raw or cooked vegetables without sauces or butter or margarine

fruits and vegetables— fresh, frozen or canned with no sugar or syrup added

dried beans and peas, including split peas, chick-peas, soybeans, lentils, baked beans and beans. (Since dried beans and peas are high in protein and low in cholesterol, they can be substituted for meat, except for certain essential amino acids)

beverages include tea, coffee, carbonated drinks

DESSERTS & SNACKS HIGH IN CHOLESTEROL

commercial pies

pastries

whipped cream

ice cream

cookies
cake
puddings
cocoa butter

fried foods
snack foods
(coconut)
(potato and corn chips)

if prep w/ oil w/chl.

DESSERTS & SNACKS LOW IN CHOLESTEROL
(high in calories, however)

home baked pastries
  and pies (made with
  non-fat milk, liquid
  polyunsaturated oil
  and egg whites)
commercial gelatins
honey, marmalade
imitation ice cream
  (made with low-fat
  milk)
nuts

cookies, cakes and
  puddings made with
  unsaturated oil and
  non-fat milk
(sherbet, ice milk)
jelly, jam
angel food cake, yellow
  cake (made with egg
  white only)
(pure peanut butter)

Boiling, baking, roasting and broiling are recommended so that the fat can be discarded. When frying use only oil high in polyunsaturates like safflower, sunflower or corn oil and never reuse the oil, since it hardens and becomes partially saturated.

8

LONGEVITY & THE SEVEN DEADLY S's

THE SEVEN DEADLY S's

There is little doubt that our genes play a considerable part in our life span. Unfortunately, there is little we can do to change our genetic structure, even with the miracle of genetic engineering. Someday, perhaps, the longevity gene will be available. You may be able to schedule a gene implant on your own chromosomes, depending, of course, on your hospital coverage.

Enough of mere idle speculation. Let's talk about today and what you can do to assure yourself of a healthier, happier, longer life. There are at present many known negative factors which adversely affect the quality, and in many cases, the quantity of our lives. I'm sure that you've heard about many of these negative health factors; however, you've probably never seen them all listed in a series such as this. The fact that they all start with the letter S is mere coincidence and makes them easier to remember.

The Seven Deadly S's are actually adverse or negative factors affecting your health. The avoidance or exclusion of them from your daily living combined with the *DR.'S F*A*S*T* 3-DAY DIETWALK®* will help to give you a head start toward good health, and a happier, longer life.

1. SALT

One of the most serious medical problems facing Americans today is **hypertension.** There are approximately 35 million people in the United States suffering from high blood pressure—or 1 out of 8 adults. Because many people are unaware of the existence of hypertension, they do not seek medical treatment for this condition. Since it rarely gives symptoms in the early stages, it is commonly called the **silent disease.** Hypertension, however, can cause serious complications such as heart attack, stroke, or kidney disease.

Hypertension can be controlled not only with medication but with a decrease in **salt** intake. With the reduction of salt to approximately 5 grams daily, we are able to reduce the blood pressure in many susceptible individuals. How do you know if you're one of the susceptible people? You don't! Some recent studies indicate that anywhere from 18–25% of people have a genetic pre-disposition to developing high blood pressure if they use excess salt. The only safe thing then that we can do is to have our blood pressure checked regularly, and stay away from salt.

The excessive use of salt in the average American diet is the result of an **acquired taste** for salting foods rather than an actual need for salt in our bodies. The first question my patients usually ask is "won't food taste bland without salt?" Our taste buds gradually adjust to a decreased amount of salt in the diet, and after a short period of time excessively salted food has an unpleasant taste. Food actually tastes better without salt.

Salt, or sodium chloride, is an essential chemical compound necessary for life. However, it is a **poten-**

tially deadly substance if we get too much of it in our diets. The fact is that it is almost impossible to develop a dietary deficiency of sodium since our diet contains more than 5 grams of salt daily, and that's in fresh unsalted food only. In the average American diet with processed foods, canned foods and salted food snacks, we consume approximately **10–15 grams** of salt a day. Actually we only need ½ **gram** of salt a day to prevent a sodium deficiency in our bodies.

How does this much salt get into our diets? First of all, salt is used world-wide as a **preservative** in many foods. It is also an essential ingredient in the **canning process.** The salt content of **processed foods** adds 5 additional grams of salt daily to our diets. There is salt, of course, in potato chips, pretzels, pickles, tomato sauce, TV dinners, crackers, tuna fish, sardines and even peanut butter. However, did you also know that there is considerable salt in cheese, butter, margarine, bread, tomato juice, ketchup, beer, soda and most breakfast cereals? Add to that the 2 grams of salt we pour every day on our meat, soups, salads, eggs and vegetables and we're getting 12–15 times more salt than we actually need to sustain life.

This excess salt intake can actually cause a **rise in blood pressure** by disturbing the kidneys' ability to eliminate this salt in the urine. The excess accumulation of sodium in the blood causes the body to retain more fluid and this **increases the volume of blood.** The heart subsequently has to work harder to circulate this additional volume of blood and high blood pressure can result from this disturbance. This is a temporary condition, if the high salt intake is decreased. However, with a continued excess salt intake, the rise in blood pressure is substantial and may become permanent. **Strokes** and **heart attacks** are the complications which can result from prolonged untreated high blood pressure.

Reduce the amount of salt used in your cooking or baking. Do not add salt to any food at the table. Use herbs, spices and condiments instead of salt. Decrease the consumption of processed foods, canned soups and vegetables, prepared meats and cheeses, bouillon cubes, salted crackers, cereals with high salt content, worcestershire and soy sauce; garlic, onion, celery and seasoned salts. Increase the amount of fresh or frozen vegetables and use unsalted margarine. Be careful of over-the-counter cold and headache remedies which may have sodium as part of their content. Avoid pretzels, potato chips, peanuts, pickles, crackers and most packaged snack foods.

Increase foods with high potassium content since these seem to have a beneficial or protective effect on hypertension. Some foods rich in potassium are oranges and orange juice, grapefruit and grapefruit juice, bananas, raw tomatoes, potatoes, squash, cabbage, broccoli, chicken, turkey and lean beef.

Remember to follow your physician's advice and recommendations in the treatment and control of high blood pressure. You may be able to control your blood pressure without the use of medication but only under a physician's supervision. Have your blood pressure checked regularly. Also check with your doctor before using any of the "salt substitutes."

You can get a booklet called **"Sodium Content of Foods"** by writing to the Office of Governmental and Public Affairs, U.S. Department of Agriculture, Room 507A, Washington, DC 20250.

Always check the label and choose a comparable food item with the lower salt content.

2. SUGAR

1. Heart Disease

Dr. John Yudin, of the University of London, recently stated that excess sugar consumption is statistically related to the development of atherosclerosis and heart attacks. The average consumption of sugar per person in England is approximately 120 pounds per year (2.3 pounds/week), and in America it may be as high as 170 pounds per year or 3 pounds of sugar eaten every week.

The discovery of methods to refine sugar from sugar cane and sugar beet in the last century has made sugar one of the most common ingredients in our everyday diets. Sugar not only is present in your sugar bowl as visible sugar, but it is a common ingredient in most products found on supermarket shelves. Of course, there is considerable refined sugar in cakes, candies, pies, ice cream, jellies, soft drinks, gelatin desserts, cookies and most desserts. However, how many of you know that there is a good deal of refined sugar in salad dressing, vegetable juices and soups?

Many investigators feel that the dramatic rise in heart attacks in Western countries in the past half century is directly related to an increase in sugar consumption. Other researchers feel that the statistical increase in heart attacks is related to both the increased consumption of refined sugar, and saturated fats. Still other investigators believe it is the increased amounts of **serum triglyceride** (one of the blood fats), which comes from eating too much sugar, that leads to heart disease. Whatever the mechanism involved, there can be little doubt that the use of too much refined sugar and saturated fat in the diet leads to an increased risk of heart attacks.

2. Diabetes

In the normal person, all carbohydrate foods (starches and sugars) and approximately 60% of all protein foods are turned into a sugar called **glucose.**

This sugar travels in the blood to the body's tissues and cells to be used as a source of energy.

Diabetes is a disease wherein the body is unable to handle sugar properly. This leads to a build-up of glucose in the blood (high blood sugar). The symptoms and signs of diabetes are: excessive thirst, excessive urination, fatigue, weight loss, vision changes and, in untreated persons, coma and death. Anyone can become diabetic, even without a family history of the disorder.

According to Dr. T.L. Cleave and other researchers, the development of diabetes is directly related to the excess consumption of refined sugar in certain susceptible people. They believe that eating excess concentrated refined sugar stresses and strains the **pancreas** (the organ which produces insulin to control the blood sugar). Initially, this stress causes the pancreas to produce too much insulin, which drops the blood sugar rapidly and in many cases causes symptoms of **low blood sugar** or **hypoglycemia.** Eventually, however, the pancreas gets tired and sort of wears out from this continued bombardment of sweets. This results in not enough insulin being produced to cope with the increased amounts of sugar eaten, and we get a high level of sugar in the blood (**diabetes**).

Diabetes, like hypertension, is also related to the accelerated development of **atherosclerosis** (hardening of the arteries) with the subsequent development of heart and vascular disease.

3. Obesity

Refined sugar provides nutritionally deficient calories which have been stripped of all nutrients (vitamins, minerals, and amino acids), and are essentially **"empty calories."** Excess consumption of refined sugar not only can lead to heart disease and diabetes, but to **obesity** and **poor nutrition** as well.

Dr. T.L. Cleave in his book, "The Saccharine Disease," stated that the primary cause of obesity was the overconsumption of refined carbohydrates. When sugar is refined, it is in a very concentrated form. For example, the calories in a heaping teaspoon of sugar are almost the same as those in an apple. It is then simple to see how easy it would be to overeat foods primarily made with refined sugar before the appetite is satisfied, as compared to overeating, for example, apples.

Obesity, like hypertension and diabetes, also has associated with it an increased risk of developing **heart disease.** Obesity is also statistically related to the development of **diabetes** and **hypertension.**

4. Dental Disease

The excess consumption of sugar promotes **tooth decay** and **periodontal disease** (pyorrhea) in both experimental animals and humans. Refined sugars tend to be trapped in tiny crevices in the enamel or between the teeth due to their minute size, and promote the formation of bacteria causing gum disease and tooth decay.

3. SATURATED FAT

We have discussed this thoroughly in Chapter 7; however, it is essential that we again mention this **Deadly S.** As you already know it is important to cut down on **saturated fats** since they elevate the blood cholesterol which leads to **atherosclerosis** and can add to the risk of high blood pressure, heart, and vascular disease.

Dietary cholesterol is an important factor in the development of coronary heart disease. **Saturated fat** may have as strong an effect on raising blood cholesterol levels as does dietary cholesterol itself. Consequently, the saturated fat in marbelized beef may be as dangerous as the cholesterol in eggs. One must keep in mind, however, that both the **dietary cholesterol** and the **dietary saturated fats** are both very important factors which elevate blood cholesterol and contribute to the development of **atherosclerosis.**

Elevated levels of blood fats have been incriminated as risk factors in the development of **cardiovascular disease.** In particular, blood cholesterol has been incriminated in the narrowing of the coronary arteries which supply the essential nutrients and oxygen to the heart muscle itself. Once these **cholesterol plaques** narrow the coronary arteries to a point where the blood supply is unable to pass through, then the individual develops a heart attack. **High fiber** and **low saturated fat/cholesterol** diets are one of the mechanisms involved in the prevention or treatment of elevated blood fats and the subsequent development of atherosclerosis.

To reduce the blood cholesterol levels we have to increase the amount of fruits and vegetables in our diet and decrease the amount of fatty foods. By increasing fruits, vegetables, fish, skimmed milk, low fat dairy products, poultry and beans in our diet we will most certainly reduce the blood cholesterol. Foods that are high in saturated fat and cholesterol and should be avoided are meats, whole milk products and eggs in particular. The best treatment for high blood cholesterol is a diet which is low in **calories, saturated fat** and **cholesterol.** This diet is currently accepted by the **American Heart Association.**

OTHER DISORDERS THOUGHT TO BE DUE TO EXCESS FAT IN THE DIET

1. **COLON CANCER:** There have been recent studies that show the excess consumption of saturated fat has been statistically related to the development of

cancer of the colon. The increased amounts of **bile acid** in the intestines may act as cancer causing agents. Also there is recent epidemiological evidence that shows the risk for developing colon cancer is significantly increased in groups of people that consume diets both low in fiber and high in fat. This finding is based on chronic exposure of the colon to high levels of bile acid that accumulate in the colon from chronic constipation.

2. **GALLSTONES:** Excessive fat intake may also overstimulate the gallbladder and aid in the formation of gallstones. Excess fatty acids, especially **saturated fatty acids,** may enhance the production of cholesterol leading to oversaturation of the bile which results in cholesterol gallstones.

3. **OBESITY:** Fat has the highest calorie density, more than twice the amount of calories as the same weight of carbohydrate and protein and is a factor in the development of obesity. For every one gram of fat ingested, **nine calories** are taken in, compared to only four calories per gram of protein or carbohydrate.

4. **BREAST CANCER:** Breast cancer may result from the increased circulation of hormones which are absorbed from the intestinal tract. This rate of absorption seems to be accelerated by fat in the colon. When estrogens (female hormones) are absorbed from the colon, they can have a stimulating effect on breast tissue. Excess fat in the intestine may allow these hormones to be absorbed at a greater than normal rate.

5. **PROSTATE CANCER:** A recent report issued by the national Academy of Sciences stated that several medical studies showed that the incidence of prostate cancer was higher in men who consume high fat diets.

4. SPIRITS

DID YOU KNOW THAT:

1. **Alcohol** is the most **abused drug** in the United States, and the 3rd cause, indirectly, of all deaths every year.
2. Approximately 15% of all people who drink will have become permanently **addicted** to alcohol.
3. **250,000 Americans** have died because of **drunk driving** in the past 10 years. That's 5 times the number of United States men that were killed in Vietnam.
4. Over one-half million **serious injuries** result every year from drunk driving.
5. More than one-half of all **traffic fatalities** (car occupants and pedestrians) are caused by drunk driving.
6. The leading cause of death in the **16–25 age group** is fatal drunk driving crashes.
7. On any weekend night, **one** out of every **10 drivers** is drunk.
8. **Drunk driving** causes more injury and deaths every year than all of the robbers, murderers, rapists and muggers lumped together.
9. Over **60%** of all murders, rapes, muggings, stabbings, shootings and beatings occur under the influence of alcohol.
10. More than **50%** of deaths from fires, drownings, suicides, accidental poisonings and home accidents and fights occur from alcohol abuse.

Now, if you're lucky enough to survive these alcohol related deaths and injuries, we'll discuss what alcohol does to you personally, and how it slowly **destroys** every living tissue and cell in your body.

One of the most dangerous characteristics of alcohol is its extremely high level of **toxicity**. Alcohol directly affects the **brain** and **liver** and indirectly affects almost every other **organ** and **tissue** in the body. One important note should be made here and that is that some people are affected more than others when small amounts of alcohol are ingested over a long period of time; however, everyone is always affected adversely when large amounts are taken over a prolonged period of time. The following summary of **complications of alcohol abuse** will give you some idea of the widespread profound effects of alcohol on your body.

1. Liver

a. **Alcoholic hepatitis:** results in jaundice (yellowish discoloration of eyes and skin), weight loss, loss of appetite, fever and liver enlargement. This condition, usually the first stage of alcoholism, may result after a relatively short period of heavy drinking (1–2 years).

b. **Fatty liver:** usually occurs after 4–5 years of chronic alcohol abuse and causes symptoms of weakness, loss of appetite, fatigue, impotence, and loss of menstrual period. The liver cells first become replaced by fat and then begin to die.

c. **Alcoholic cirrhosis:** this is the final stage of alcohol abuse. The liver and spleen enlarge, blood spots appear on the face and hands, the breasts enlarge (in males) and the testicles shrivel up. In this stage, the muscles waste away, the legs and abdomen swell, the kidneys begin to fail, and progressive weakness, weight loss and jaundice occur. The final stages include mental confusion, disorientation, coma, and death.

2. Nervous System

a. **Neuritis:** (inflammation of nerves) approximately 25% of alcoholics develop neuritis of the legs.

The symptoms include loss of feeling, numbness and tingling in the legs and occasionally the arms.

b. **Nerves behind Eye:** become affected with symptoms of blurring of vision and may progress to blindness.

c. **Brain and Spinal Cord:** their nerve fibers are directly affected by alcohol. The early symptoms include loss of memory, disorientation, apathy and confusion. These progress to loss of muscle coordination, decreased sensation of touch, eye muscle paralysis and psychosis. The final stages are hallucination, convulsions, coma and death.

3. **Heart:** Heart disease directly related to chronic heavy drinking is being seen with increasing frequency. It usually occurs in people under the age of 50 and is thought to result from direct damage to the heart muscle by alcohol. The death rate from this type of alcoholic heart disease is well over 45%, usually caused by an irregular heartbeat which results in heart failure.

4. **Pancreas:** Acute inflammation of the pancreas may result after a relatively few bouts of heavy drinking. It usually is seen in younger alcoholics and **can be fatal** after the first attack. Symptoms include: severe abdominal pain, vomiting, rapid heartbeat, fever, chills and weakness. If not treated promptly, it may progress to bleeding into the pancreas, loss of calcium from the body, kidney failure, shock and eventually death.

5. **Intestinal Tract:** Inflammation of the stomach and peptic ulcer occur in over 25% of alcoholics. One of the most common life-threatening complications from chronic alcoholism is swelling and bleeding from the veins in the esophagus. This condition results in massive hemorrhage (bleeding) and kills approximately 18% of all alcoholics.

6. **Infections:** Because of malnutrition and weakened defense mechanisms, the alcoholic is subject to many infections which would not ordinarily affect the

nonalcoholic. Pneumonia is the most common complication resulting in the death of an alcoholic. The infections which they get frequently include: tuberculosis, kidney, blood, heart and brain infections.

And if all this isn't enough to scare you, then consider this—alcohol has more calories (7 calories per gram) than most foods on a weight basis and it is one of the most serious hazards to any successful diet program. The additional calories which are consumed in the American diet from alcohol have been shown to contribute to approximately 25% of overweight problems.

5. SMOKING

DID YOU KNOW THAT:

1. Cigarette smoking is now the **major single cause of cancer deaths** in the United States, according to the latest report of the Surgeon General.
2. Smoking is the largest **preventable cause of death** in the United States.
3. Smoking each year causes:
   a. 250,000 deaths from **heart disease**
   b. 80,000 deaths from **lung cancer**
   c. 20,000 deaths from **chronic lung disease**

4. **One** out of every **5 cancer deaths** is caused by smoking.
5. A 1–2 pack a day smoker has a life expectancy **7–10 years shorter** than a non-smoker.
6. Cigarette smoking increases the risk of developing **lung cancer** 10 times that of a non-smoker.
7. Smoking during **pregnancy** may cause miscar-

riage, still born, mental retardation, growth defects and premature births.

8. Low tar, low nicotine cigarettes are not safe. In fact, some studies show that low tar cigarettes may actually give a higher content of carbon monoxide in the blood which is dangerous to the heart muscle. **There is no such thing as a "safe cigarette."**

9. The most effective way to stop smoking is—**"DON'T START."** If you do smoke, ask your doctor about the best way for you to stop. If your doctor smokes, get another one!

10. If you smoke and stop smoking, you will **gradually increase your life expectancy** year after year. After you've stopped for **10 years,** your risk of death from any cause is the same as a person who never smoked. **GOOD NEWS!**

Cigarette smoking is implicated in the development of **cardiovascular disease** and has been shown to statistically increase the chances of having a heart attack 3 to 6 times over the non-smoker. In fact, cigarette smoking probably is one of the most important risk factors for **coronary artery disease.** The nicotine and carbon monoxide levels in the blood will increase the heart rate, constrict the blood vessels, and elevate the **blood pressure.** In addition to the coronary artery disease and high blood pressure caused by cigarette smoking, **lung cancer** and **chronic obstructive lung disease** are two more complications, accounting for over 100,000 deaths per year.

Smoking decreases the **HDL-cholesterol** (good cholesterol) levels in the blood and thereby eliminates one of the body's protective mechanisms against the development of coronary heart disease. Smoking also has a dangerous effect on the vascular system by narrowing the blood vessels due to their constriction by

nicotine and causing the blood vessel walls to be irritated and therefore more readily to accept plaques of cholesterol. High levels of blood **carbon monoxide** which are found in smoking also have an adverse effect on the circulation and heart by decreasing the amount of oxygen that the blood cells carry.

A national health and nutrition survey conducted from 1976 through 1980 studied approximately 11,000 people 15 to 74 years of age. Nearly **80% of smokers** compared to nonsmokers were found to have potentially dangerous levels of carbon monoxide in the blood, which can increase the chances of heart disease, in addition to the development of lung disease. A regular **walking** program decreases the amount of carbon monoxide and increases the oxygen content in the blood stream. Both of these factors lead to a decreased desire to smoke and illustrate how walking can help you "kick the habit."

6. STRESS

A study by the **Presidential Science Advisor** in 1977 called stress a major problem affecting the lives of millions of Americans. Stress has been implicated in causing a wide array of physiological and psychological disorders. The sources of stress are multiple, ranging from marital problems, bereavement, financial problems, overwork, job insecurity, personal relationships, family situations, work related stress, etc. This list of stresses that we are bombarded with daily is almost endless.

We all are aware that there are a number of **common stress-related disorders** that affect all of us. Among them are tension headaches, menstrual irregularities, backaches, upset stomachs, over-eating, diarrhea, loss of appetite, insomnia, and occasionally, palpitations. Stress is also a component in many more **serious disor-**

ders such as migraine, colitis, peptic ulcer, angina, high blood pressure and heart disease.

STRESS KILLS DESPITE HEALTHY DIET

In a recent study conducted at the Bowman Gray School of Medicine, it was reported that **social stress** may lead to **hardening of the arteries** and **heart disease** even among those on **healthy diets.** Two groups of monkeys were fed low cholesterol, low fat diets for 22 months. One group of monkeys lived in a stable environment, whereas the second group was placed in an unstable setting. The group in the stressful environment developed severe hardening of the arteries compared to the monkeys in the stable setting, even though both groups were fed the same diet.

Stress in susceptible people activates the body's **sympathetic nervous system** which causes the blood vessels to constrict. This narrowing of the blood vessels leads to a temporary elevation of the **blood pressure.** There is also an increased level of **hormones** secreted by the sympathetic nervous system when we are under stress. These hormones cause the **kidney** to retain extra fluid which has an additional blood pressure raising effect.

These changes described above are only temporary responses made by the body to stress situations, and the blood pressure returns to normal after the stress is gone. However, after prolonged periods of stress, **structural changes** begin to occur in the blood vessels and kidneys. These changes, if pronounced enough, could possibly lead to a permanent rise in blood pressure (**hypertension**) even after the stress has passed and you are perfectly relaxed. Hypertension increases the risk of **heart attacks** and **strokes.**

HOW TO DEAL WITH STRESS

It seems simple to say then, "avoid stress." However, in practice it is very difficult. We are subjected to stresses every day at work and at home. Just when we think we can relax, another stressful situation comes up. How then are we to deal with a condition over which, in most cases, we have little control? The answer, then, is not in eliminating stress, but in learning effective ways to deal with it in our everyday lives.

According to Dr. Herbert Benson of the Harvard Medical School in Boston, the use of **relaxation techniques** can result in a significant decrease in blood pressure. Many physiological changes result from using relaxation techniques including a reduction in heart and respiratory rates, an increase in serum norepinephrine (a chemical in the blood which tends to give a feeling of well being), and a significant decrease in the systolic and diastolic blood pressures. He describes his relaxation techniques as sitting in a comfortable position, closing your eyes, concentrating on relaxing each muscle group, and repeating a phrase or word of the individual's choosing with each exhalation (letting out your breath).

Other methods of coping with stress include regular sleep, good diet habits, leave job tension at work, take breaks from stressful situations, talk about frustration with co-workers and family, leave family problems at home when you're at work, cultivate a hobby and don't overwork yourself to the point of fatigue. Drink less coffee, tea and colas since caffeine is a stimulant and increases stress. Eliminate alcohol and nicotine since both lower the body's resistance to stress. Learn to recognize your own stress level (headaches, palpitations, fast heartbeat, insomnia, etc.) so that you can begin to cope with it early.

Many people rely on tranquilizers and sedatives to relieve tension; however, the effects of these drugs are short-lived. The worst way to deal with stress is to sit still and wait for it to disappear. Never try to fight stress—stress always wins! The best way to combat stress is to get out and **walk away from tension.** How many times have you noticed that after a long walk you feel less tense and more able to cope with your problems? This feeling of calm results from an **increased oxygen** supply and a **decreased carbon dioxide** level in your blood. Recent studies have also shown that walking increases the level of certain brain chemicals (**endorphins** and **norepinephrine**) which have a mood-elevating effect. No wonder we feel so invigorated after a **refreshing walk!**

7. SEDENTARY LIFE STYLE

WALKING SLOWS THE AGING PROCESS

In a recent Gallup poll survey of over 500 people over the age of 90 years of age, one significant finding emerged: all these individuals were physically active.

Our bodies are one of the few machines that break down when not in use. A physically active person is one who is both **physically and mentally alert.** A walking program can actually slow down the aging process and add years to our lives. Walking stimulates a healthy **circulation,** aids in **digestion,** improves **muscle tone** and **strength,** and increases the **oxygen** utilization by all the tissues and cells of the body.

Individuals who lead inactive lives seem to often experience deterioration in both their mental faculties and their muscular systems. Inactivity leads to depression, frustration, general weakness and the loss of many physical abilities. **Regular exercise** is one of the best ways to release much of this energy and emotion and can lead to a more physically active and alert individual. In our society, unfortunately, older people have been led to believe that the retirement years are the time to become physically inactive.

Nothing can be further from the truth. Being retired does not mean being inactive. Actually, this is the time of our lives when activity is more important than at any other time. The more active you are, the less likely you are to be plagued with the debilitating diseases of aging. Remember, it is never too late to begin an exercise program, even after years of inactivity. **The body responds to exercise at any time.**

PREVENTIVE MEDICINE

Medical care spending has increased to 9.4% of the Gross National Product. The American health-care system has concentrated all of its attention to the treatment of disease and not nearly enough to its prevention. If people were educated to the principles of preventive medicine, there would be a tremendous reduction in many of the so-called degenerative diseases that affect our modern civilization.

According to Dr. William Cannel, Professor of Medicine, Boston University School of Medicine, **obesity control** appears to be a major factor in the control of many major chronic illnesses. According to Dr. Cannel, if all Americans were at their ideal weight, there would be **35% less heart failure and stroke** and **25% less coronary heart disease.** He stated that weight reduction is an ideal treatment for hypertension, diabetes, gout and degenerative arthritis, combined with standard medical therapy.

The **DR.'S F*A*S*T* 3-DAY DIETWALK®** is presently one of the most important weapons that we have in the long-term fight against obesity and its life-threatening complications. This diet and exercise program can be a significant factor in the prevention of many health problems and degenerative conditions of aging that affect all of us, including the endless battle of the bulge. The *DR.'S F*A*S*T* 3-DAY DIET-*

WALK® is a unique program enabling you to lose weight, stay thin, keep fit and live longer all in one easy-to-follow, inexpensive, effective package. At last a diet that's as good for your figure as it is for the rest of you. The essential points to remember are:

1. **Walk** at least 60 minutes **3 days** per week or 30 minutes every day except Sunday.
2. Increase the **fiber** content of your food.
3. Decrease the total amount of **cholesterol** in your diet.
4. Avoid the **7 Deadly S's** (Salt, Sugar, Saturated Fat, Spirits, Smoking, Stress, and Sedentary Life Style).

GOOD LUCK!

9

STAY FIT & TRIM WITHOUT KILLING YOURSELF

FITNESS FALLACIES

1. **Exercise turns fat into muscle. False!** When you exercise you are actually burning fat; however, this fat does not turn into muscle. What actually occurs is that the fat passes from its storage depots and goes into the bloodstream where it is taken to the muscles to be used as fuel. As the amount of fat in the body decreases, the muscle size appears to increase.

2. **Weight-lifting strengthens the heart muscle. False!** Lifting weights actually strengthens and builds your muscles but not your heart, since this is an anaerobic training exercise, not an aerobic one. The only exception to this is when you are using light weights and working out along with aerobic exercises; then you can actually strengthen the heart muscle.

3. **If you are thin, you are physically fit. False!** When you are thin, you do not necessarily have to be physically fit. Physiologically, fitness refers to the efficiency of the heart and lungs to take in oxygen and distribute it through the body in an efficient manner.

Only a lifetime exercise program can guarantee physical fitness, in particular cardiovascular fitness.

4. It is necessary to take your pulse during and after exercise. False! It is not necessary to take your pulse during exercise since the body physiology has a fail-safe mechanism which first causes a sighing respiration when your pulse has exceeded 120 beats per minute. Also gasping for breath or shortness of breath is an indication that you are going too fast. It is not necessary to push your heart rate up to any astronomical figure in order to gain fitness. A steady exercise program, guaranteed in walking, will raise the heart rate 30 to 40% above the resting heart rate. This moderate increase is more than sufficient over the long-term, to increase the oxygen uptake and delivery to all the body's tissues and cells. If you become tired or fatigued, stop and rest.

5. The resting pulse rate is a good indicator of physical fitness. False! In many cases a slow pulse rate, as found in professional athletes, is a good indicator of physical fitness; however, the pulse rate is affected by many factors and the resting pulse rate should not be used as a guarantee for good physical fitness. The **recovery pulse rate** is a reasonable indicator of physical fitness. This is obtained by taking your pulse immediately after exercise and then retaking your pulse two minutes after exercise. If the pulse rate has slowed by 25 to 30 beats per minute then you are in reasonably good shape; however, if your pulse rate has not slowed to this extent, then you are probably not in good physical condition. This indicator is not 100% true and other factors have to be taken into consideration also, such as your heart and lung capacity and the circulatory system.

6. Vigorous exercise daily provides the best physical fitness. False! Studies have shown that regular continuous exercise in the form of a moderate intensity exercise such as walking on an every-other-day basis provides the same physical fitness development as a strenuous exercise program on a daily basis. Vigorous exercise is not essential, since the same physiologic, cardiovascular and fitness-conditioning benefits occur with walking, without the potential dangers and hazards of strenuous exercise.

WALKING AS AN EXERCISE

Walking remains the **safest, most effective** form of **exercise** known to man and woman. With all of the hazards of jogging and competitive sports, you may wonder why anyone would participate in so violent an exercise as jogging. Well, the answer is simple. We live in a masochistic society and we have been conditioned to believe that an exercise or activity has to be painful in order for it to be beneficial. For instance, how many of us have attempted to diet with vigorous starvation diets to obtain a thin figure, engaged in back-bending exercises to have a well-conditioned trim body, or suffered a painful sunburn to obtain a beautiful tan?

The simple, basic, medical, scientific fact is, **exercise does not have to be painful** in order to have beneficial results. **Walking** produces the same, let me repeat, the same **physiological, psychological,** and **weight-control** benefits as jogging and other strenuous type exercises without the hazards. The **cardiovascular** benefits are exactly the same without the strain.

The medical journals are filled with studies about the health **benefits of walking** and they also are filled with an equal number of reports regarding the **hazards of jogging** and other strenuous exercises. Remember, you can achieve better health and fitness without stress and strain and inconvenience and—let me point out to you—a walking program is the only exercise that you can safely carry out for the rest of your life. **Walking is the road to a healthier, happier, longer life.**

WALKING: THE PERFECT AEROBIC EXERCISE

Aerobic exercises include walking, swimming, cycling, dancing and other active sports. This type of exercise is designed to increase endurance and fitness and is brought about by the action of the large muscle groups (leg, thigh, hip, back and chest muscles) allowing a continuous supply of oxygen to course through these muscles. The increased supply of oxygen brought about by aerobic exercise causes calories to be burned at a faster rate as we have seen in Chapters 1 and 2. This aerobic exercise also improves the efficiency of the **cardiovascular system** and is considered to be a significant factor in the **prevention** of **heart** and **vascular diseases.**

Aerobic exercise is defined then as the type of exercise where the oxygen demand of the large muscles of the body does not exceed the oxygen supply. This type of aerobic exercise usually occurs in constant, sustained exercise such as **walking,** but not in strenuous high-intensity exercises (jogging) where the oxygen demand exceeds the supply, causing a condition known as **oxygen debt.**

In order for aerobic exercise to promote **cardiovascular fitness,** it must be done at least every other day and its duration must be at least 20–45 minutes of continuous activity. It is definitely not necessary to increase the heart rate to a level 60–80 percent higher than the normal resting heart rate in order to develop cardiovascular fitness. Walking at a comfortable pace may increase the heart rate 30–40 percent above your normal resting heart rate, and this is more than adequate to improve the oxygen delivery and the oxygen uptake to all the body's cells, tissues and organs. This process is a gradual one and occurs over a period of many months.

Recent research has once and for all dispelled the myth that animals, including humans, use more energy to run than to walk an equal distance. Using treadmill studies, physiologists have shown that you use the same number of calories per distance regardless of whether you walk or run. In other words, you **burn no more calories running one mile** than you do **walking the same mile.** What's the hurry!

The following walking program (Fig. 3) illustrates that cardiovascular fitness and weight loss will occur over a gradual period of time without resorting to strenuous exercises or marathon events. With all the possible hazards of running—why run when you can walk. So it may take a little longer—better to be safe than sorry. **Slow and steady wins the fitness race.**

The following chart (Fig. 3) represents a training program for physical fitness development with men 40–57 years of age, for a period of 20 weeks. These men walked for 40 minutes, 4 days a week, and their increased physical fitness and weight loss was equal to a 30 minute, three-day per week jogging program, with men the same age.

LACK OF EXERCISE IS RISKY

According to the U.S. Department of Health and Human Services, the American lifestyle is typified by passive forms of entertainment and by the almost total elimination of physical labor from most daily activities. The average American spends between 40 to 50 hours per week watching television and the average American child spends more time in front of the television set than he does in the classroom. Only 1 percent of the energy used in factories, industries and farms is supplied by human muscle, when just a century ago up to one-half of the energy was supplied from human labor. The conversion to a mechanized, industrial society has led to serious health defects. Physical inac-

FIGURE 3

Effects of walking on physical fitness of middle-aged men

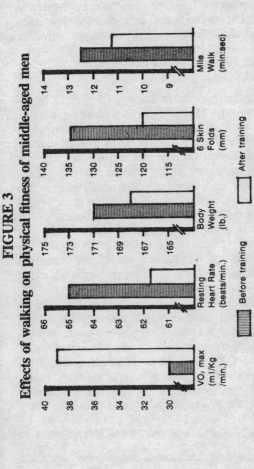

VO₂ max—Maximum oxygen uptake (aerobic capacity). Body weight—Determined by underwater weighing technique. Skin folds—Body fat determined by skin folds measurements

Reprinted with permission of The Physician and Sportsmedicine, a McGraw-Hill publication, from an article "How Much Exercise is Enough?" by Michael L. Pollock, Ph.D., June 1978.

tivity is one of the main contributing factors in obesity and its related complications. It is also related to a lack of flexibility, strength and mobility in most people, especially the elderly. Inactivity has been implicated in the development of heart and lung disease, low back pain, elevated cholesterol and high blood pressure.

HOW MUCH EXERCISE IS SAFE AND BENEFICIAL?

In a recent study reported in Lancet, the British medical journal, nearly **18,000** British middle-aged male civil service workers were studied for more than **eight years.** The findings indicate that there was an inverse relationship between the level of **activity** and the development of **coronary artery disease** and its subsequent morbidity and mortality. The levels of exercise reported in this study consisted of active recreational activity or the home environment type of exercise activity. The main point brought out by this study is that the training effect which is obtained from regular dynamic aerobic exercise of a **moderate intensity** can both improve the health of the individual and reduce his risk of **coronary artery disease.**

The question no longer is whether or not to exercise, but the main issue is **how much exercise is both beneficial and safe?** As seen by the above study, **moderate low intensity regular activity** provides benefits of reduced risk of heart disease. Repetitive activities which use large muscle groups such as walking, swimming, bicycling, aerobic dancing, and rope skipping all provide moderate low intensity type exercise.

THE FALLACY OF JOGGING FOR FITNESS

When exercise first became a subject for scientific investigation and research, it was **walking** that was studied, not running.

Studies conducted in the early 1950's by Professor J.N. Morris, a British researcher, involved walking as an exercise and its role in the **prevention of heart disease.** Professor Morris found that studies conducted on postmen and bus conductors revealed that those who walked suffered fewer fatal heart attacks as compared to those who remained seated.

This statistical correlation has been repeated constantly by numerous scientific studies over the past 30 years. This finding was recently underlined by a study at the Stanford University School of Medicine by Dr. Ralph Paffenbarger; the results showed that an activity which burns approximately 300 to 350 calories daily resulted in a markedly decreased incidence of heart disease. A **brisk walk** for **one hour daily** burns approximately **350 calories** and has been shown to be the **ideal exercise** for the greatest number of people over the longest period of time.

If walking is such an excellent, safe exercise, then why should one bother to engage in more strenuous activities such as jogging? There are some researchers who believe that if the exercise is more vigorous, it places a more strenuous demand on the heart and other organs so that the body is more prepared to deal with stress. Many other researchers, on the other hand, feel that this is sheer nonsense. By stressing and straining the body's vital organs, including the muscles and skeletal system, there is no indication that this strengthens these particular organs to prevent them from being damaged by future stress. In fact, the statistics have been more than adequate to stress the point that strenuous exercise such as jogging or running in the average individual results in more **bodily injury** than one could hope to be able to compensate for by the possible prevention of disease.

THE MEDICAL BENEFITS OF WALKING AS AN AEROBIC EXERCISE

1. Improving the transport of **cholesterol** through the body in a way to prevent accumulation and injury to the blood vessel walls. Also by decreasing the amount of blood fats (cholesterol and triglycerides) circulating in the body.

2. Improved receptivity of the body cells to **insulin** which means a smoother utilization of blood sugar and the reason, perhaps, for the improvement in diabetics controlled by a program of regular exercise.

3. Increasing a group of hormonal chemicals in the body called **endorphins** which seem to have a mood elevating and tranquilizing effect, helping to reduce stress and tension.

4. Improved **lung efficiency and capacity** and **breathing techniques** which help to improve the quality of life among asthmatics and individuals with lung disease.

5. Improvement in the overall **circulation** of the blood by increasing the volume of blood and the amount of oxygen carried by the red blood cells.

6. Beneficial effects on the **vascular system** by dilating (opening) the arteries and allowing more blood to flow through them; and by squeezing the leg and abdominal veins by the muscles used in walking to aid in the return of blood to the heart.

7. Lowering the **blood pressure** by dilating (opening) the arteries, making the blood vessels more flexible and elastic and by lowering certain chemicals (catecholamines) in the blood that elevate the blood pressure. All of these factors decrease your chances of getting a heart attack, stroke or kidney disease.

8. Promoting **weight loss** and assisting in **weight control** by directly burning calories and by indirectly controlling your appetite.

9. Protecting the **heart** by improving the return of blood from the leg veins, decreasing the risk of blood clot formation, improving the flow of blood through the heart's own coronary arteries and by increasing the amount of HDL (GOOD-CHOLESTEROL-SUB-MARINE) in the blood which protects the heart against fat accumulation.

10. Improving the efficiency of the delivery and uptake of **oxygen** to all of your body's cells, tissues and organs, thus promoting a longer healthier life.

HOW TO STAY FIT & LIVE LONGER

Walking has a tonic effect on both the body and the mind. It is the simplest, most basic of all our daily activities and as a regular program of exercise, it can actually slow the aging process. As we walk through city or country our blood supply is effectively squeezed back through the veins of our legs into the heart and then recirculated into the general circulation, bringing increased amounts of oxygen and nutrients to all our body tissues and cells. This increased **oxygenation** is the basis for deterring or slowing down the aging process.

Researchers at San Diego State University showed that a correlation existed between **reaction time** and **aging**. The results indicated that reaction time decreases with age, with one exception. Older people who exercised regularly did not suffer this usual slow-down in reaction time. They also noted that there seemed to be a correlation between reaction time and cardiovascular health (Medicine & Science in Sports, Vol. II, No. 2, 1979).

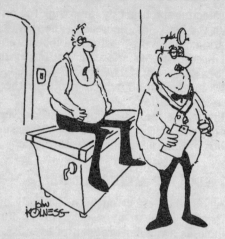

Used with permission of *Family Practice News*, March 26, 1982 and John W. Kolness

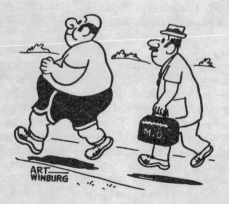

Used with permission of *Medical Tribune*, Jan. 27, 1982 and Art Winburg

EXERCISE AND THE AGING PROCESS

Exercise is certainly not the fountain of youth; however, a regular exercise program may protect you from some of the ravages of aging.

1. **Heart:** Like the other muscles of the body, as we age the heart may become weakened so that it is unable to pump as much blood through the blood vessels to the body with each beat as it had done in years past. Studies have shown that exercise can **strengthen the heart muscle** and again minimize or decrease the effects of aging by continuing to enable the heart to pump blood at a regular rate.

2. **Blood Vessels:** When your heart contracts, the major blood vessels dilate or widen to absorb the flow of blood. As you grow older, your blood vessels may lose some of their **elasticity** and since the vessels do not expand sufficiently when the heart contracts, your **blood pressure** rises. Exercise has been shown to help keep these blood vessels flexible and, therefore, can prevent a rise in blood pressure which is often associated with aging.

3. **Lungs:** Regular exercise helps to condition the **muscles of respiration** (chest wall and diaphragm) to work more efficiently. Exercise also assists in opening more **usable lung space** and thus improves the lungs' efficiency in extracting oxygen from the air we breathe.

4. **Muscles of the Body:** As we age, muscles can also lose their elasticity which results in a slow reaction time. With a regular program of exercise, the **muscle fibers** can be strengthened and the elasticity preserved, thus improving reaction time, especially in motor functions such as driving an automobile.

5. **Skeletal system:** The **bone strength** and **structure** which depends primarily on its **mineral content** is

aided by exercise. This is thought to be due to the muscular pull on the bones exerted by exercise. Aging causes a loss of minerals from the bone. This condition, commonly called **osteoporosis**, seen primarily in post-menopausal women, weakens and thins the bones. Exercise appears to have a beneficial effect on this condition, and has also been noted to alleviate the symptoms of certain types of arthritis.

JOGGING IS HAZARDOUS TO YOUR HEALTH

Americans have been brought up on the pain-pleasure principle. In order for something to be good for you it must either taste bad (ex. medicine) or it must hurt first (ex. exercise) before it can be beneficial. The jogging craze that started over the past decade was a prime example of this masochistic tendency. Never before had so many people engaged in such a dangerous sport. The complications resulting from jogging are being seen by physicians with increased frequency.

The following list summarizes many of the complications resulting from jogging that have been reported in the medical literature. While many of these jogging injuries are relatively common, others are extremely rare. However, the fact remains that these complications from jogging do indeed occur, and can be avoided by utilizing a walking program. Walking, incidentally, produces the same physiological, psychological, cardiovascular fitness and weight control benefits as running, with virtually no risk at all. Walk, don't run!

POSSIBLE COMPLICATIONS RESULTING FROM JOGGING

Muscular System: Muscle cramps, pulls, sprains, and tears; ligament and tendon injuries; cartilage tears. These usually affect the foot, ankle, knee, thigh, hip and back.

Skeletal System: Stress fractures (small bones of feet, long bones of leg, and, rarely, pelvis, hip, and spinal vertebrae). Also slipped discs and arthritis flare-ups.

Nervous System: Pinched or compressed nerves in the neck and low back resulting in pain and numbness in the arm or leg (sciatica). Also compulsive behavior (running mania) and depression have been reported.

Metabolic System: Heat exhaustion, chemical imbalances in the blood (ex. potassium loss) and, rarely, heat stroke.

Immune System: Itching and redness of skin; hives and swelling of face and neck; and, rarely, anaphylaxis (shock, swelling, irregular heartbeat).

Gynecology: Menstrual irregularities, infertility, miscarriages, hormonal imbalances and, rarely, birth defects and prolapse (dropping) of the urinary bladder & uterus.

Renal System: Protein and blood in the urine, and, rarely, kidney damage caused by decreased blood supply and dehydration.

Cardiovascular System: Palpitations, chest pain, heartbeat irregularities and, rarely, heart attacks and sudden death.

Respiratory System: Shortness of breath, fatigue, wheezing, and, rarely, exercise-induced asthma, and partial lung collapse.

Gastrointestinal System: Abdominal cramps, bloating, nausea, vomiting, and, rarely, stress ulcers and bloody diarrhea (caused by decreased blood supply to the colon).

The Eye: Mild irritation, conjunctivitis, and, rarely, vitreous hemorrhages and retinal detachments.

Environmental: Frostbite, heat exhaustion, dogbites, auto & bike accidents, and, rarely, lung damage from polluted air (ozone and high levels of carbon monoxide).

10

HOW TO GET BACK INTO YOUR CLOTHES

BEAUTY BENEFITS OF WALKING

Every time you start out on your daily walk, literally thousands of changes occur in your body. Your **blood volume** and **red blood cells** increase, your **heart rate** becomes faster, your **lungs** enlarge taking in and absorbing more oxygen, your **muscles** expand and contract, your **energy** level increases, and your **nervous system** becomes less tense. The results of these activities will certainly go to make a **stronger, trimmer figure.**

Your general appearance will be noticeably improved following your daily walk, since the walk will definitely improve your **digestion** and **circulation** and enable you to ease away tension. Many people have noted a better night's **sleep** and disappearance of those **stress lines** around your eyes. Walking also can enable you to have better **posture** and a better **figure** following the changes previously noted.

Your **complexion** will improve with walking since

160

there is nothing better for the complexion than the increased blood circulation to the skin. We have even noted that walking has shown improvement in **acne** programs when combined with medical treatment.

Muscle tone certainly is one of the most important results for which we are looking. After your daily walk you will notice that your muscles will be toned and firm and that after you have been on your walking program for some time, you will notice many of the fatty bulges and deposits decreasing in size. Your **stomach** will flatten and your **calves** and **thighs** will become more trim and the **buttocks muscles** will become more proportioned. Many of these changes are due to improved muscle tone and secondarily to the strengthening of the spine.

We have noted in many studies that the circulatory system can increase the amount of oxygen, not only to many parts of the body but even to the **hair.** Many of us who have lackluster, dry hair will notice an improvement after a walking program. The hair, because of the increase in protein from the improved metabolism secondary to increased blood flow, will gain more life. It will become glossier and appear healthier.

Walking, therefore, is as **natural** as breathing and as helpful as an adequate night's sleep. Walking not only trims you down, but firms up your muscles. Walking is actually the only non-strenuous exercise that is relaxing, healthy and beautifying, and can be part of a regular program of **health** and **beauty care.**

Remember, it is not necessary to kill yourself in order to stay fit and trim. Walking produces the same figure control and aerobic fitness benefits as jogging and other strenuous exercises without the potential dangers. The fact remains that exercise does not have to be painful in order to be effective and beneficial.

THE MYTH OF CELLULITE

Cellulite is a different kind of fat requiring special types of treatment to get rid of it. **False!** Fat is fat, and cellulite is actually a **myth.** When fat cells immediately beneath the skin enlarge, sometimes the strands of fibrous tissue that connect these fat cells don't stretch. This gives ordinary fat a lumpy appearance on the hips and thighs and has been given the mythical name— **cellulite,** by gimmick diet promoters.

In a recent study conducted at Johns Hopkins University in Baltimore, fat biopsies (small pieces of tissue) were taken from people with lumpy fatty tissues (the mythical cellulite) and from people with regular fat deposits. The result: all of the biopsy specimens were identified under the microscope as **ordinary fat cells.** There was no tissue identified as cellulite!

Any product claiming to be a special treatment designated to get rid of "cellulite" is phony. The Food & Drug Administration has recently published a booklet entitled "Cellulite," in an effort to protect the public from spending money for a magical cure for a mythical disorder. Write to the Consumer Information Center, Dept. 560K, Pueblo, CO 81009 for a free copy of this booklet.

PHYSICAL EFFECTS OF A WALKING PROGRAM

The following physical and physiological effects will be noted after you have been on your walking diet for a six-week period:

1. **Flatter stomach**—the abdominal muscles will be firm and support the intra-abdominal contents so that the appearance will be of a flatter stomach.

2. **Slender thighs**—leg strengthening and loss of

fat in the thigh muscles will reduce the outer and inner thigh dimensions.

    4. **Firmer buttocks**—the large buttocks muscle, called the gluteus maximus, will contract and draw the buttocks higher and make them appear firmer.

    4. **Upper arms leaner and shapelier**—the muscles of the upper arm, which include the triceps and biceps, will increase their tone and the fat loss from the fleshy part of the upper arm will combine to form a firmer, shapelier arm.

    5. **Firmer, higher appearing breasts**—the pectoral muscles of the chest will lift the breasts to make them appear larger although they will not actually grow in size.

    6. **Increased level of energy**—with increased aerobic training, the lungs, heart, and circulation will be improved in efficiency and add more energy to your day.

    7. **Improved nightly sleep**—a regular walking program will aid in sleep without the use of sedatives or tranquilizers.

ON A CLEAR DAY YOU CAN WALK FOREVER

Most of us do not realize that we walk more than **125,000 miles in an average lifetime,** which will take us approximately 5 times around the entire earth. Walking is a complex physiological and bio-mechanical process of getting from one place to another—the act of **locomotion.** Walking involves hundreds of muscles, thousands of nerves, and many bones, joints and ligaments to produce a near perfect bio-mechanical method of locomotion, involving the synchronous movement of the legs and arms.

    The **rhythm of walking** involves a steady pace which will become automatic and the brain will regulate the length of your stride, your heart rate, oxygen uptake and other physiological adjustments. You should concentrate on making smooth even steps, avoiding spurts of speed and abrupt changes in pace. The energy expenditure over your walking period will remain constant and your walk should leave you feeling relaxed, with effortless motion. Colin Fletcher, author of **THE COMPLETE WALKER,** said it best when referring to rhythm: "an easy unbroken rhythm can carry you along hour after hour, almost without your being aware that you are putting one foot in front of the other."

The **speed of walking** should be between 2½ and 3½ miles per hour since walking is a moderate type exercise. If you increase the speed beyond 4 miles, the upper arms and shoulders swing too fast and the lower leg muscles have to work too hard to compensate, thus producing wasteful energy expenditure. It is important that you walk at a comfortable speed, one that does not leave you breathless. This type of walking activity falls into the **aerobic** form of exercise in which you are taking in **oxygen** as fast as you are burning it up. This is an efficient use of energy. **Anaerobic,** on the other hand, is the opposite condition which is caused by an over-exertion of muscles (e.g., running fast) working beyond their capacity. This type of anaerobic exercise leads to the buildup of **lactic acid** in the muscles causing pain, discomfort and fatigue, a condition known as **oxygen debt.**

The **gait of walking** refers to the motions of your legs, feet and arms during the phases of walking. Most of the energy required for walking is provided by the muscles and joints of the ankles, knees and hips (Figs. 4 and 5). When we overstride or understride, we disrupt the natural walking gait. An easy steady, unbroken stride will produce the rhythm and gait necessary for the effortless act of walking. Also, it is necessary to avoid toeing in or out during the walking gait, since this wastes energy. Try to concentrate on keeping your toes straight and thus your stride will be even and rhythmic. During the act of walking, your arms swing naturally from the shoulders. Overswinging the arms purposely during walking will reduce the efficiency of the act of walking and subsequently tire you early during your walk. If you don't try to concentrate on the act of walking during your rhythmic stride, you will actually allow the muscles to relax and perform more efficiently.

FIGURE CONTROL

Your body burns calories all the time (**basal metabolic rate**) no matter what you are doing. Even when you are sleeping, between 50 and 85 calories an hour are expended during sleep. This is why it takes a certain amount of calories daily just to maintain your body weight. Therefore, it is obvious that if you are actually doing something in the form of physical activity or exercise, you will burn up more calories than the basal metabolic rate, which only involves sedentary activities like sleeping, eating and sitting.

Remember that with **walking** you increase the **aerobic capacity,** which is the body's ability to take in more oxygen through the lungs, dissolve it into the blood stream, and pump it more efficiently so that it circulates to all the muscles and cells of the body. This **oxygen** is used to produce **energy.** As this oxygen burns off fat, you will have a **trimmer, leaner figure.**

As surprising as it sounds, **walking** is the most **reliable** and **safest** way to lose excess fat and flab. Crash diets and fad diets may do a faster job, but they usually are dangerous, exhausting, monotonous and debilitating. It is also noted that people who take off weight on rapid weight reduction programs put the weight back on just as fast as they took it off. **Weight reduction**

Figure 4
The Inferior Extremity

Left: Movements of the inferior extremity. Lateral view showing direction of movement in flexion of thigh, leg, foot, and toes.

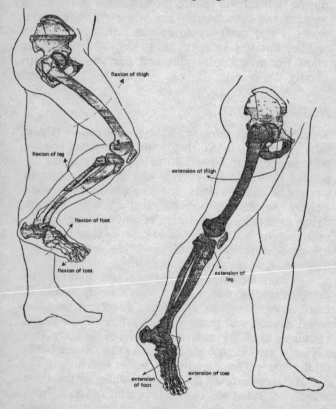

Right: Movements of the inferior extremity. Lateral view showing direction of movement in extension of thigh, leg, foot, and toes.

With permission of McGraw-Hill from *Concise Anatomy* by L.F. Edwards and Gaughran, McGraw-Hill, 3rd ed. 1971. Drawing by Thelma Frazier.

Figure 5

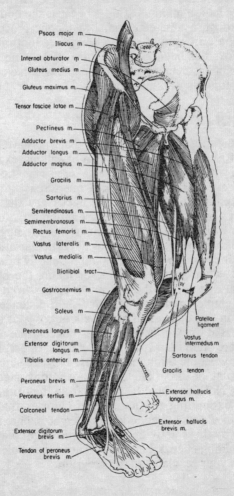

Psoas major m.
Iliacus m.
Internal obturator m.
Gluteus medius m.
Gluteus maximus m.
Tensor fasciae latae m.
Pectineus m.
Adductor brevis m.
Adductor longus m.
Adductor magnus m.
Gracilis m.
Sartorius m.
Semitendinosus m.
Semimembranosus m.
Rectus femoris m.
Vastus lateralis m.
Vastus medialis m.
Iliotibial tract
Gastrocnemius m.
Soleus m.
Peroneus longus m.
Extensor digitorum longus m.
Tibialis anterior m.
Peroneus brevis m.
Peroneus tertius m.
Calcaneal tendon
Extensor digitorum brevis m.
Tendon of peroneus brevis m.

Patellar ligament
Vastus intermedius m.
Sartorius tendon
Gracilis tendon
Extensor hallucis longus m.
Extensor hallucis brevis m.

Reproduced by permission of Oxford University Press from *Essentials of Human Anatomy* by Russell T. Woodburne, 6th Ed. 1978.

through walking is a more gradual process and the most important point to note is that the chances of regaining fat are minimal. This is because the body has gone through a time-consuming metabolic process in which the adjustment to the weight reduction and weight loss has been gradual. Subsequently, **no rapid weight gain** has been noted with people who have been on a continuous walking program.

HOW FAR DO I HAVE TO WALK?

One of the most important things that you have to be aware of is that in order to begin a walking exercise program you do not have to be an exercise fanatic. You do not have to be a jogger or a quarterback for the Philadelphia Eagles. It is only necessary that you maintain a regular walking exercise program.

You will see that there are many ways to augment your walking program by walking at particular times of the day or evening when you would ordinarily ride. For example, when you are driving or taking the bus to work, park or get off the bus a few blocks from your place of employment and walk that short distance. For lunch, you can take a half hour walk out of your lunch break, and at work or home you can concentrate on the stairs more often than you use the elevator or escalator.

Many people think that because they are active all day at home or in the office, they are getting adequate exercise. Nothing could be further from the truth. You are not expending the number of calories that are needed in a weight reduction or weight maintenance program by these activities. There is no doubt that you are expending energy, but you will need to supplement this with your **regular walking program.**

MAINTENANCE WEIGHT & FIGURE CONTROL WALKING PROGRAM

Your walking program will consist of a **one-hour walk 3 days per week** or a **½-hour walk every day except Sunday.** You may choose the schedule that suits your own daily routine. If you decide on the 3 day per week schedule, you may choose any 3 days of the week that suit you the best.

1 HOUR 3 DAYS PER WEEK:

If you decide on the **one hour 3 days per week schedule,** you don't have to walk for one hour continuously. Twenty minutes morning and night, to and from work, for example, and twenty minutes at lunchtime, give the same results as walking one full hour at a time. Also two ½ hour walks during the day are equally effective (**TABLE VI**).

½ HOUR EVERY DAY EXCEPT SUNDAY:

If it's easier to walk **½ hour every day except Sunday,** the health, fitness and weight-loss benefits are the same, as long as you walk consistently. Remember, the beauty of a walking program is that, with a little planning, you can "fit" it into your own schedule—as it can help you to **"fit" comfortably into your clothes.** (**TABLE VI**).

WALKING SPEED:

As previously shown in **TABLE I,** there are **three walking paces** (slow, moderate and fast). The fast-pace walk of 4 mph is too strenuous and exhausting for a weight-loss walking program. You may find that your pace (miles per hour) falls somewhere between the moderate and slow paces. A **brisk** but not too fast walk is usually about **3 mph (moderate pace).** If this is too

fast and tiring for you, then cut back to a slightly slower
pace, until you are comfortable and not out of breath,
or excessively fatigued. On the **MAINTENANCE
WEIGHT & FIGURE CONTROL WALKING PRO-
GRAM** you should walk for one hour **3 days** every
week or ½ hour daily except Sunday. This program is
based on consistency and not on speed.

WALKING DISTANCE:
   How far should you walk in an hour or a ½ hour?
Don't worry, it's the **TIME** and not the distance which
is important. Whether you walk 2, 2½, or 3 miles in one
hour; or 1, 1¼, or 1½ miles in one-half hour, you will
still benefit from your walking program. As long as you
are consistent in the time you walk every day, the
distance that you travel is unimportant.

HAPPY WALKING!

MAINTENANCE WEIGHT & FIGURE CONTROL WALKING PROGRAM

TABLE VI

1. 3-DAY PER WEEK WALKING SCHEDULE

Week Day	Time	Distance Slow Pace (2 mph)	Distance Moderate Pace (3 mph)
EVERY MON.	60 minutes	2 miles	3 miles
EVERY WED.	60 minutes	2 miles	3 miles
EVERY FRI.	60 minutes	2 miles	3 miles

2. EVERY DAY EXCEPT SUNDAY WALKING SCHEDULE

Week Day	Time	Distance Slow Pace (2 mph)	Distance Moderate Pace (3 mph)
EVERY MON.	30 minutes	1 mile	1½ miles
EVERY TUES.	30 minutes	1 mile	1½ miles
EVERY WED.	30 minutes	1 mile	1½ miles
EVERY THURS.	30 minutes	1 mile	1½ miles
EVERY FRI.	30 minutes	1 mile	1½ miles
EVERY SAT.	30 minutes	1 mile	1½ miles

11

PEDAL POWER: SHAPE-UP/SLIM-DOWN

INDOOR SHAPE-UP/SLIM-DOWN PROGRAM

How many of us have the luxury of living in a temperate climate for twelve months of every year? Not many! Does this mean we have to give up **THE DOCTOR'S F*A*S*T* 3-DAY DIETWALK®** because of inclement weather? Absolutely not!

Most of us gain our *winter weight* because of forced inactivity, even if our calorie intake stays the same (which it usually doesn't). The combination of more calories and less activity leads to more unwanted pounds. The average weight gain per person from Thanksgiving to early January is approximately three to six pounds all across America.

How often have you remarked, however, after a vacation that you're surprised that you didn't gain as much weight as you thought? You certainly ate enough! The reason is simple: you WALK more in one week on a vacation than you probably do in a month at home. This is why you cannot afford to give up your walking program for even one day, let alone a week or a month. Don't let winter-wind, summer-storms, hail, sleet, ice and snow "fatten you up for the kill"—your heart and lungs need to be taken for a walk each and every day, otherwise they may decide to stop walking, too!

As with our outdoor walking program, an indoor program which involves the rhythmic, repetitive use of the body's large muscles when sustained for a moderate period of time also provides *aerobic fitness* or cardiovascular training. Remember, you will also **burn calories** with your indoor shape-up/slim-down program as you walk or pedal away those extra pounds.

INDOOR WEIGHT-LOSS WALKING PROGRAM

If the weather is such that your walking program has to be discontinued for a day or two, then we have to turn to our home-exercise program. It is essential that you have a regular schedule to follow since the key to any successful program, which includes our daily walking program, is **consistency.**

1. WALKING IN PLACE:

Walking in place is an excellent indoor exercise. You can expend the same number of calories, lose the same amount of body fat, and strengthen your heart and lungs as if you were walking outdoors. With this method you should move your arms briskly and lift each leg two to three inches from the ground. A rate of approximately 50 to 60 steps per minute (count only when the right foot hits the ground) should allow you to complete your walking requirements for the day in **30 minutes.** You may break this up into three **10-minute sessions** each day in order to prevent fatigue.

A retired physician wrote to me recently about a novel idea that he uses for indoor walking in inclement weather. He has 2 TV sets at opposite ends of a 30 foot recreation room, and walks up to an hour a day (divided into three 20 minute sessions) back and forth without missing any of his favorite shows. By using a pedometer he was surprised to find that he walks about 2½ miles in this hour. Talk about walking in comfort!

2. LIGHT RUNNING IN PLACE:

Light running in place is not detrimental to the back and legs in the same sense as jogging outdoors. The reason for this is that you are only lifting your legs off the ground momentarily and therefore the force and impact with which your foot hits the ground is not as severe as when running on a hard surface and landing with four to five times your body weight. The gradual light running in place can be done in two or three **five-minute** sessions for a total of **ten to fifteen minutes** each day, and remember to **stop if you become tired.** A rate of approximately 75–85 steps per minute is more than adequate (again remember to count only when the right foot strikes the ground) for aerobic conditioning and weight loss. You may gradually be able to build up to three **10 minute** sessions daily.

Both light running and walking in place can be combined on any given day. You also have the opportunity to watch **TV** or listen to the **radio** during this type of activity. Remember, no matter how boring this indoor exercise program is, it is an **essential part** of your walking diet and exercise program.

CAUTION:

If you become fatigued, dizzy, short of breath, or experience pain and/or discomfort anywhere, then promptly stop your exercise. Refer to **CHAPTER 12** for **MEDICAL EXERCISE TIPS & CAUTIONS.**

One of the best ways to continue your all-weather

shape-up program is by using an exercise bicycle. This type of exercise equipment is the only investment you'll ever need to make on the road towards fitness and permanent weight control.

EXERCISE BIKES

A. STATIONARY BICYCLES:

The most reliable and successful form of indoor exercise can be accomplished with the stationary bike. These basically are bicycles without a rear wheel and are mounted on a stand. They range in price from under $100 to several thousand dollars for computerized models. Important features to look for in a stationary bicycle are: a comfortable seat with good support, adjustable handle bars, a quiet pedal and chain, and a heavy front wheel. These come with speedometers to tell the rate that you are pedaling and odometers to tell the mileage that you pedal.

B. HOME-MADE STATIONARY BIKE:

During extremely bad weather, there is another way to keep up with your schedule of walking without purchasing an expensive exercise bike. The use of a **home-made stationary bike** will suffice until the weather clears. You can convert any bike in your garage into a stationary bike with the purchase of an inexpensive **"rear-bike-wheel converter"** at any sporting goods or bicycle store. It is easily attached and removed without any mechanical ability. When the weather is nice, the converter can be removed easily and your bike can be used outdoors.

The above-mentioned stationary bikes fall into the category of **aerobic exercise equipment**. Aerobic exercisers provide rhythmic continuous motion of the large muscle groups such as the arms and legs. The main benefit of this type of exercise is that the heart and lungs must work harder than normal to supply these large muscle groups with **oxygen**. During regular sustained aerobic exercise, your heart and lungs will become more efficient. Aerobic exercise also **burns a significant quantity of calories** and is an essential part of your weight-loss program. Remember that increasing the strain and stress on your heart by increasing the work load lever or dial is not essential for aerobic fitness. In most cases it is not necessary to increase the work load lever beyond minimal tension or zero.

The **STATIONARY BIKE** is the **safest** type of indoor exercise equipment that can be purchased to supplement your walking diet program. Either the stationary bike or walking/running in place can be used in inclement weather or at times when outside walking is inconvenient. This type of indoor exercise can be utilized with music, TV, telephone, or even reading (a bookstand attachment can easily be clamped to the handle bars, leaving the hands free). All this luxury and convenience while you are exercising those unwanted pounds away. What could be simpler! Remember, exercise does not have to be painful and uncomfortable to be beneficial. An inexpensive stationary bike works just as well as an expensive one.

Pedaling at a comfortable rate of **10–15 miles/hour** will complete your daily maintenance exercise requirements in **30 minutes** (divided into three 10-minute sessions to avoid fatigue). Consult the chart for the exercise bike-conditioning program before using your stationary bicycle.

NOTES:

1. Tension Control level set at zero tension.
2. Time and miles per hour are approximate.

CALORIES BURNED ON YOUR INDOOR SHAPE-UP/SLIM-DOWN PROGRAM

I. WALKING IN PLACE (3 mph)
1. Each 10 minute session   = 50 calories burned
2. Three 10 minute sessions daily = 150 calories burned
   (30 minutes)

II. LIGHT RUNNING IN PLACE (5 mph)
1. Each 10 minute session   = 75 calories burned
2. Three 10 minute sessions daily = 225 calories burned
   (30 minutes)

III. STATIONARY BIKE (12 to 15 mph)
1. Each 10 minute session   = 100 calories burned
2. Three 10 minute sessions daily = 300 calories burned
   (30 minutes)

Remember, everytime you burn up 3,500 calories, you will lose 1 lb. of body fat. The results are cumulative, which means you simply add up the number of calories burned day by day until you reach 3,500 calories. It doesn't make any difference how long this takes (10 days, 15 days, 30 days, etc.). The result is always the same—**you lose 1 lb. of body fat.**

---

3. Stop at the first indication of fatigue, shortness of breath, or pain and/or discomfort anywhere (see **CAUTIONS LIST** on next page).
4. Follow conditioning chart for gradual weight loss and physical fitness. Do not attempt to set endurance or speed records.
5. The above chart can be used to supplement, complement, or replace outdoor walking program, depending on weather.

10 WEEK CONDITIONING PROGRAM FOR STATIONARY BIKES WITH SPEEDOMETERS

Weeks	Total Time Per Day (Min./Sec.)	Divided Into 3 Sessions of (Min./Sec.)	Distance Total (Miles)	Speed (mph)	Frequency (Days) Per Week	Weight
1	3:45	1:15	5/8	10	5	
2	3:45	1:15	7/8	15	4	
3	7:30	2:30	1¼	10	5	
4	7:30	2:30	1⅞	15	4	
5	15:00	5:00	2½	10	5	
6	15:00	5:00	3¾	15	4	
7	22:30	7:30	3¾	10	5	
8	22:30	7:30	5⅜	15	4	
9	30:00	10:00	5	10	5	
10	30:00	10:00	7½	15	4	

MAINTENANCE SCHEDULE

	30:00 min.	10:00 min.	5 to 7½ miles	10 to 15 mph	4 or 5 days	

6. If you are already finished with your outdoor conditioning walking program, you may be able to follow the daily maintenance program without going through the conditioning program. Use your own judgment and level of physical fitness to determine this.

7. If you have not completed your outdoor walking conditioning program, use common sense and your level of physical fitness to determine which week you will begin with on above chart. If it is too tiring, then move back to an earlier week.

8. You may alternate days of outdoor walking and indoor cycling or you may even divide each day into half outdoor and half indoor exercise. The program is completely flexible.

9. Follow list of cautions (on next page) carefully.

10. Be sure to exercise regularly for maximal physical fitness and weight loss.

CAUTIONS IN THE USE OF A STATIONARY EXERCISE BIKE

1. First and foremost, always get a **complete physical examination** from your physician before engaging in any exercise program.

2. Individuals with **back, knee or hip problems** should be exceptionally cautious before using an exercise bike and should check with their physician first.

3. People with certain forms of **heart disease** may not be permitted to use an exercise bike and should check with their physician.

4. Caution should always be used when **moving your exercise cycle,** as with any heavy, bulky

object. Never attempt to move the exercise bike up or downstairs yourself.

5. Do not use the exercise bike immediately before going to bed as the exercise may tend to keep you awake.
6. Do not use the exerciser immediately before or after eating or drinking.
7. Be sure that the exercise bike is on a sturdy, level floor, and be careful when mounting and dismounting the bike.
8. Exercise should be stopped promptly if you develop shortness of breath, a rapid heartbeat, palpitations, pain or discomfort anywhere or any unusual symptom. Consult CHAPTER 12 for medical precautions.
9. Wear a good, sturdy shoe or sneaker when pedaling (never pedal barefoot).
10. Be sure there is adequate ventilation in the room or area that you use your exercise bike in. If the room gets too warm, your heart rate may go up very rapidly without your being aware of this fact.

TIPS ON PURCHASING EXERCISE BIKES

1. Before purchasing an exercise bike, get on the bike in the store and try it out.
2. Make sure that the seat is comfortable and wide enough.
3. Make sure that the seat adjustment is adequate so that you can adjust the height to the length of your legs.
4. Your knee should be bent only slightly at the bottom of the stroke. (If your knees are bent too much, then you will put too much strain on them.)
5. Models which have bike handles which move

in conjunction with the pedals are worthless (your body is only going along for the ride).

6. Models which have a **lever** which allows you to work your upper body along with the pedaling action are not necessary and they may put too much stress and strain on the back and neck muscles.

7. Be sure that the **spokes** on the bike wheel are covered with some form of covering (metal) especially if there are small children around who could stick their hands into the moving wheels.

8. The **tension device** usually comes on most bikes and is of no real importance. Set it at zero or minimal tension.

9. The only accessories that are essential are a **speedometer** to indicate your speed and an **odometer** to record mileage.

10. Make sure that your bike has a **chain guard** to prevent your pants or trousers from getting caught while pedaling. (If this is not present, make sure you roll up your trouser leg.)

OTHER TYPES OF EXERCISE EQUIPMENT

There are many other types of indoor exercise equipment that can be purchased and used effectively. However, most of these are extremely costly, difficult to use, bulky to store and have many disadvantages not found with the stationary bike. The following types of equipment are listed here for your review.

1. **TREADMILL:** A treadmill is a type of conveyor belt which is supported by a steel frame. They come in both motorized and non-motorized varieties and unfortunately they are extremely expensive, running between $300 and $1,500. They are extremely large and difficult to store and they have been noted to cause ligament and muscle strain injuries.

2. **MINI-TRAMP:** These are miniature trampolines which are called rebound exercisers. They stand three or four feet wide and are approximately six inches off the ground. They run approximately $150 to $200 and can be used almost anywhere in the home. One of the advantages of these mini-trampolines is that they reduce the shock or trauma to the feet and ankles when jumping up and down. However, there are many disadvantages to this type of exercise apparatus. They include falls from loss of balance, ankle strains or sprains from twisting, head injuries from bouncing too high and hitting an overhang, and back injuries from twisting.

3. **ROWING MACHINES:** The main disadvantage of rowing machines is that they are strenuous and are really designed to develop upper body strength, not cardiovascular fitness. These machines also can be dangerous to individuals who have high blood pressure or heart disease because they are not true aerobic exercises.

4. **JUMP ROPES:** The main advantage of jump ropes is that they are the least expensive of all the indoor exercise apparatus and can be used just about anywhere in the home. Among the disadvantages noted with this type of activity are that they can induce falls by tripping and the repetitive jumping on a hard surface can be traumatic to the feet and ankles.

5. **PASSIVE EXERCISE MACHINES** (Belt Vibrators, Roller Machines, Whirlpool Baths and Vibrators): These so-called exercise devices contribute next to nothing in the development of cardiovascular fitness. They are not aerobic exercises and have no place in an exercise and diet program. Women who have a tendency toward varicose veins, when using roller machines, have frequently had small blood vessels break under the skin causing hemorrhages. Belt vibrators have been implicated in jarring internal ab-

dominal organs with occasional damage to these vital structures.

6. **PROGRESSIVE-RESISTANCE EXERCISERS:** In this category we have to include weights, springs, pulleys, and many types of elastic devices. This type of exercise, in contrast to aerobic exercise, stresses the stimulation and strengthening of the large muscles of the body. These machines do very little for the heart and lung capacity and do not increase the consumption of oxygen; subsequently, they are not useful in fitness conditioning, nor in burning calories to help you to lose weight. Many of these progressive-resistance exercises can be dangerous and have been known to cause elevation of blood pressure in susceptible persons.

12

WALKING WEIGHT-LOSS TIPS

BEGINNING YOUR WEIGHT-LOSS WALKING PROGRAM

In the beginning of your weight-loss walking program, pick a terrain that is level since hills place too much strain on your body. Concentrate on maintaining **erect posture** while walking. Walk with your shoulders relaxed and your arms carried relatively low with natural motion at the elbow. When you hold your arms too high as in running, your neck and shoulder muscles become stiff and tired. Walking should be at a **brisk** (moderate pace 3 mph) pace; however, if you get out of breath, then you're probably walking too fast. Remember to stop when you are tired and then begin again after resting. Begin slowly and gradually increase your walking time each week. Remember, it is the **time** and not the distance that you walk each day that is important.

CONTINUING YOUR WEIGHT-LOSS WALKING PROGRAM

Exercise programs for weight control and cardiovascular fitness have one thing in common. They have relatively **high dropout rates.** This results from a multitude of factors, such as physical strain and discomfort, psychological changes, breaking old habits, complexity and duration of the programs, and general boredom and monotony. **Regular walkers,** however, continue their exercise programs because they **feel better** and **enjoy walking.** Many people regard exercise as a painful process; walking, however, is not the least bit uncomfortable because it is a natural non-strenuous form of exercise.

CHOOSE YOUR OWN TIME AND PLACE

The beautiful part about walking as a diet and exercise is that you aren't limited to a particular time and place. Walking is the type of activity that can be done anytime and anywhere. Homemakers can walk in the morning, right after they get the children off to school. Those employed outside the home can walk before or after work. If you drive to work, park your car a little farther away from the office, and walk the rest of the way. If you take public transportation, get off a few stops sooner and walk. If the weather is bad, an enclosed mall or shopping center could be the perfect place for your walk. Take a half hour from your lunch break and walk, especially if you're stuck indoors all day—think of how good that fresh air feels. When the weather prevents you from venturing outdoors, then get on your stationary bike and shape-up and slim down (Chapter 11).

If you plan to do most of your walking in the city, you can use your walking time to explore streets and neighborhoods you've never seen before. Plan your walks—your city or town has a guide book containing historical sites, restaurants, shops of interest, and cultural centers; walking can truly aid you in expanding your horizons. Make sure you walk in well-lit areas that are not deserted and be careful of walking alone, especially at night in unfamiliar areas. If you live near a park, the country or the seashore, a weekend walking trip will give you a new lease on life. Take time to explore the world around you; the wonders of nature are many and are literally at your feet. Each season has its own natural beauty. Enjoy them all while you walk off those extra pounds.

THE CORRECT WAY TO WALK

Walking along the street with your head down and your shoulders slouched forward, and your stomach stuck out is certainly not the correct way to walk. The most important stance in walking is to walk tall, with your head up, stomach in, and your chest out. If this is not your usual stance in walking, you may be able to correct it as you engage in your walking program.

Stride is one of the most important aspects in your walk. There is no correct single length stride. Try to stretch as much as you can when you are walking and keep your body slightly forward as you walk. It is important to thrust your legs forward and to take a longer arm swing if possible.

As far as the **pace** is concerned, never push when you are walking to a pace that will make you tired. Even if your pace is not rapid and you do not tire easily, you can consider that you are walking at a normal speed. If you do happen to get tired after a short period of time, stop and rest and then re-start again at your own pace.

The **rhythm** in walking is a type of condition that will naturally come as you begin your walking program. Let your body be loose and your stride even, and your rhythm will naturally develop. You will notice that the walking surfaces you encounter will control your pace and rhythm, especially going up or down hill.

To get the most out of your walking program, walk with the **heel-and-toe method** (Figure 6). Proper walking uses calf muscles more productively and improves blood flow to these muscles.

WEATHER CONDITIONS

I caution my patients against any kind of physical exertion when the weather is extremely hot and humid or cold and windy. There's no need, however, to stay indoors during mild to moderate changes in weather conditions, since very few of us have perfect weather all year. In fact, if you just wait for that warm, sunny, low humidity day to come along, forget it! You'll never walk. That type of day is never there when you want it. The most important consideration in your walking program is to continue it on a regular basis, day in and day out. **Consistency** is the key word no matter what the weather is except in the extreme changes of weather that we will now discuss.

RAINY WEATHER

Rain presents another of life's little difficulties and nature's way of getting your walking program all wet. Well, a light rain should never prevent anyone (providing the weather is mild) from taking his or her daily walk. A raincoat, umbrella, and rubbers should be handily stored in the glove compartment, office or home so that they can do the job that they were intended for. You'll be surprised how fresh the air feels and smells after being cooped up indoors all day. If the weather is really bad, then an enclosed mall can be the perfect place to take your daily walk.

Have you ever noticed while you were stuck in

Figure 6

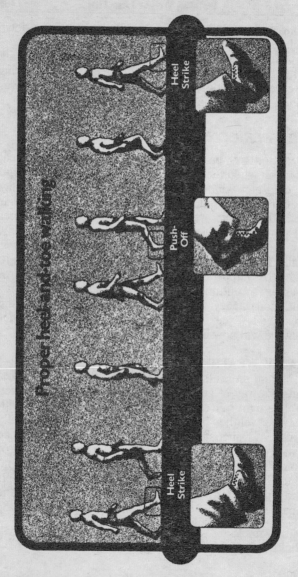

Proper heel-and-toe walking

Heel Strike   Push-Off   Heel Strike

How to walk properly

To get the most out of your walking program, walk with the heel-and-toe method. Proper walking uses calf muscles more productively and improves blood flow to these muscles. The diagram on the previous page explains heel-and-toe walking.

Heel Strike: Heel of leading foot touches the floor before the ball of the foot and toes

Push-Off: Knee is bent so heel is raised: weight is shifted forward. (This is essential and you should feel the action in the calf muscles.) Toes push off to next step.

Heel Strike: Leg is accelerated forward to get in front of body. Foot is positioned for next heel strike.

With permission of U.S.V. Laboratories, Inc., Medical Department, Tuckahoe, NY

---

rainy day traffic how comfortable and happy the walkers are as they stroll by your car with their umbrellas? They look at you and smile like you're the one that's all wet. How many times have you said to yourself, if I could just park the car and get out and walk, I'd make better time. We have become accustomed to driving everywhere, no matter what the weather is like, or how far we have to go. We never seem to have the time or inclination to walk and have developed into a society of **sedentary, overweight, wide bottomed mammals.** According to Darwin's Theory of Natural Selection we may eventually evolve into a special type of humanoid, with something resembling ball bearings on our buttocks for locomotion.

WALKING IN COLD WEATHER

The most important consideration in any exercise program is to maintain it on a **regular** basis. However, when winter weather is extremely cold one should avoid exercising outdoors when conditions are **hazardous.** Walking in the **snow** can be dangerous because you can never tell what type of terrain is underneath the snow cover and injuries are sustained quite easily. Also, **icy** conditions should be avoided since the danger of slipping and injury are always present. There are many good alternatives to continue your walking program on an indoor basis which we have discussed in Chapter 11. If, however, the conditions are such that you feel that you would like to continue your walking program in cold weather there are several precautions that we must mention.

WINTER WALKING PRECAUTIONS

1. If you have any type of **medical condition** (heart, lung, kidney, diabetes, high blood pressure, etc.), you should avoid winter walking.

2. If you develop any **symptoms** such as shortness of breath, dizziness, fatigue, or pain and discomfort anywhere, promptly discontinue winter walking.

3. Follow **medical precautions** outlined at the end of this chapter.

4. **Dress properly** and make sure that you wear extra layers of clothing, heavy **sweatsocks** or **thermal socks,** a **face or ski mask** may be a good idea, and **mittens** or **ski gloves** are helpful. Mittens keep the fingers together and provide more warmth than regular gloves. Make sure that the **layered clothing** that you wear is loose fitting and can be easily adjusted so that you have the ability to open all layers if necessary. If you begin to perspire, you should be able to partially

open your clothing so that the perspiration can evaporate. It is interesting to note that you can get up to 100 times as cold in sweat-soaked clothing than in dry clothing.

   —**Shoes**—a lined shoe or boot will be particularly helpful in preventing numbness of the toes and feet and will help to preserve the circulation by preventing heat loss.
   —**A scarf** over your mouth will warm the air before it is inhaled.
   —**A hat** will also preserve body heat.

   5. **Wind**—Take special precautions with winter wind. Start your walk into the wind, since you should face the worst part of the weather while you are still dry and relatively fresh. If you start your walk first with the wind at your back, you might get overheated and perspired and then when you return and walk into the wind, the perspiration could freeze on your skin with the possibility of developing **frostbite.** Cases of **hypothermia** (the body's inner temperature dropping below normal) have occurred in conditions such as this where the wind chill factor was such that its effect on a heated perspiring body produced hypothermia which is a dangerous condition.

   6. **Visibility**—It is important to realize that in the winter visibility may be poor and the possibility of auto accidents is increased. Be sure that you wear highly colored clothing, especially if you are out after dark, and be sure that you pick a well-traveled route where the automobile traffic is limited.

WINTER WEIGHT LOSS WALKING

   Since winter is the time that most of us usually gain weight, a winter's walk can not only be fun but actually has an added **slimming effect** for you as a bonus.

   Walking in cold weather has all the benefits of

walking in warm weather with one basic plus—you don't have to walk as long or as far to get the same benefits, in particular the same weight loss benefit. Since there is more exertion involved when you walk in cold weather, calories are expended more rapidly. Studies show that while a one hour walk at 3 miles per hour (moderate pace) burns approximately 350 calories per hour, the same walk on a cold winter day expends close to **400 calories per hour.** Therefore, you can accomplish the same benefits and weight loss with only a **¾ hour walk** as compared to the one hour walk in a temperate climate. The basic physiological facts behind this result from the added weight of your clothing necessitated by the cold weather and the subsequent extra effort needed in walking. The result: **MORE CALORIES BURNED PER MINUTE.**

HOT, HUMID WEATHER

Hot and humid weather has its own special set of circumstances. Generally, you have the option in hot or humid weather of being able to avoid these weather extremes by just changing your walking times to early morning or after sunset to avoid the hazards associated with heat and humidity.

When the temperature is above 75°F or if the humidity is above 60%, there is the danger of not being able to cool the body off. As we exercise, we expend energy and produce heat. The only effective way to dissipate that heat is by the evaporation of sweat from the body surface. Since this process is impaired by **high temperatures** and **high humidity,** the body temperature will rise. **Radiant heat** from the sun will also increase the body temperature. Even with adequate fluid intake before and after exercise in hot weather, it is still a strain on the cardiovascular system. A walk in the early morning or late evening will avoid most of the problems associated with high temperatures and humidity, and radiant heat exposure.

Heat exhaustion with its rare complication of **heat stroke** can be avoided by these simple precautions. There is, however, on rare occasions, that extremely hot or humid day when it is even unbearable to walk early in the AM or the late evening. High humidity presents many difficulties with any outdoor exercise program and should be avoided whenever possible.

Here, again, are the times to quietly and peacefully turn to Chapter 11 on the indoor shape-up/slim-down program and turn up the air conditioner and relax as you burn away those unwanted pounds.

HIGH ALTITUDE

High altitude can also affect your response to exercise, since there is a decrease in the oxygen content of the air. Fatigue sets in more rapidly during exercise since the blood will be transporting less oxygen to the muscles. Caution is advised, especially if you have a pre-existing lung or heart condition. If you fatigue easily or develop difficulty in breathing, then you should stop your walking program. For most people, however, a cautious and gradual approach to exercise here will have no adverse effects.

MEDICAL TIPS AND PRECAUTIONS

1. Consult your doctor before beginning any diet or exercise program and request a complete physical examination. Follow his recommendations carefully.
2. If you are currently under a doctor's care for any medical problem, make sure your physician feels that it is safe for you to embark on the walking-diet program.

3. Start your walking-diet conditioning plan slowly. Walk for approximately 15 minutes a day for the 1st 2 weeks, then 30 minutes daily the next 2 weeks, and finally 60 minutes every other day thereafter.

4. Any time that you become fatigued, stop walking and rest. You can break your walking times into 15, 20, or 30 minute sessions if you tire easily.

5. It is not necessary to take your pulse and increase your heart rate to a rapid level in order to burn calories or develop fitness. Walk at a steady, comfortable pace so that you're not out of breath. If you're short of breath or your pulse rate is rapid then you're probably walking too fast.

6. Stop the walking-diet program if you develop any discomfort or symptoms such as headaches, dizziness, palpitations, shortness of breath, fatigue, back or leg aches, chest or abdominal pain, or any other unusual symptoms. Report these symptoms promptly to your physician. Any inflammation of the foot, blisters, calluses, corns, bunions or ingrown toenails should also be reported to your doctor if they persist or interfere with walking.

WALKING SHOES

Walking shoes should have a thick cushioned sole and heel, preferably crepe material, and should have a good sturdy shank and sole. Avoid high heels and platform shoes and especially high heeled boots. There are many excellent walking shoes on the market; however, make sure that the shoe fits properly, feels comfortable and has good support. Tennis shoes, basketball shoes, conventional sneakers, jogging and running shoes are definitely not designed for your walking program. Most of these light-weight shoes do not have the adequate support necessary for a walking program. They may also cause excessive perspiration and blisters when you walk for long distances, because of inadequate ventilation.

WALKING SHOE TIPS

1. **Flexibility:** Holding the heel of the shoe in one hand, you should be able to bend up the front end with little difficulty.
2. **Shank:** The more arch support, the better; otherwise, there is a greater tendency to develop tendinitis on the inside of the foot.
3. **Shoe Covering:** Material should be heat resistant and allow for breathability (natural substance such as suede or leather).
4. **Toe Box:** ½ to ¾ of an inch between the longest toe and the front of the shoe.
5. **The Counter:** The portion which is the raised area over the heel that helps to prevent irritation should be of a good quality with a padded lining.
6. **The Sole:** A thick resilient type crepe material is the best: the more absorbent, the better. The tread design is of secondary importance.

WALKING AND HIKING ASSOCIATIONS

Adirondack Mountain Club, Inc.
172 Ridge Street
Glens Falls, NY 12801

American Forestry Association
1319 18th Street, N.W.
Washington, DC 20036

Appalachian Mountain Club
5 Joy Street
Boston, MA 02108

Appalachian Trail Conference
P.O. Box 236
Harpers Ferry, WV 25425

The Federation of Western Outdoor
  Clubs
512½ Boylston E. #106
Seattle, WA 98102

National Audobon Society
950 Third Avenue
New York, NY 10022

National Campers & Hikers
  Association
7172 Transit Road
Buffalo, NY 14221

National Park Service
North Atlantic Regional Office
15 State Street
Boston, MA 02109

National Wildlife Federation
1412 16th Street, N.W.
Washington, DC 20036

The New England Trail Conference
P.O. Box 115
West Pawlet, VT 05775

Potomac Appalachian Trail Club
1718 N. Street, N.W.
Washington, DC 20036

Sierra Club
530 Bush Street
San Francisco, CA 94108

U.S. Forest Service
Box 3623
Information Office
Portland, OR 97208

U.S. Geological Survey
(Areas East of Mississippi)
P.O. Box 25286
Federal Center
Denver, CO 80225

U.S. Geological Survey
(Area East of Mississippi)
1200 S. Eads Street
Arlington, VA 22202

Walkabout International
Box 6540
San Diego, CA 92106

Walking Association
4113 Lee Highway
Arlington, VA 22207

Wilderness Society
1901 Pennsylvania Avenue, N.W.
Washington, DC 20036

APPENDIX
CALORIE-FIBER COUNTER

Food Item	Serving Size	Calories	Dietary Fiber (In Grams)
MILK AND MILK PRODUCTS			
Buttermilk	1 cup	88	0
Cheese:			
American	1 ounce	105	0
cheddar	1 ounce	115	0
colby	1 ounce	110	0
monterey	1 ounce	105	0
mozzarella	1 ounce	80	0
mozzarella, part skim	1 ounce	70	0
muenster	1 ounce	105	0
parmesan	1 Tbsp. grated	25	0
provolone	1 ounce	100	0
Swiss	1 ounce	95	0
Cottage cheese:			
less than 1% fat	½ cup	90	0
2% fat	½ cup	100	0
4.2% fat	½ cup	130	0
Cream, heavy, whipped	1 Tbsp.	30	0
Ice cream: vanilla	½ cup	135	0
chocolate	½ cup	140	0

Ice milk	½ cup	90	0
Milk:			
2% fat	1 cup	120	0
evaporated, not diluted	1 cup	345	0
skim	1 cup	85	0
whole	1 cup	150	0
Pudding, made with whole milk (vanilla,			
chocolate, butterscotch or banana)	½ cup	175	0
Sherbet	½ cup	135	0
Yogurt:			
plain unflavored	1 cup	140	0
plain unflavored, lowfat	1 cup	125	0
fruit varieties	1 cup	230	0

Food Item	Serving Size		Calories	Dietary Fiber (In Grams)
VEGETABLES AND LEGUMES				
Asparagus:				
boiled	4	medium spears	10	0.9
cut, boiled	½	cup	15	1.1
Avocado, fresh	½	medium	240	2.2
Bean sprouts	½	cup	5	1.6
Beets, diced or sliced, boiled	½	cup	35	2.1
Broccoli, boiled	½	cup–½" pieces	15	3.2
Brussels sprouts, boiled	½	cup	15	2.3
Cabbage, shredded, boiled	½	cup	10	2.0
Carrots:				
sliced, boiled	½	cup	15	2.3
	1	medium–7½" × 1⅛" diam.	20	2.3
raw	6	strips (1 oz.)	5	0.8
Cauliflower:				
boiled	½	cup	5	1.1
raw, sliced	½	cup	5	0.9
Celery:				
raw	1	stalk	5	0.7
raw, chopped	½	cup	5	1.1

Food	Amount	Measure		
Coleslaw	½	cup	60	1.7
Corn:				
canned, drained	⅓	cup	40	3.1
on the cob, boiled	1	ear—5" long	155	5.9
Cucumber, raw	6	slices (1 oz.)	5	0.1
	1	small—6⅜″× 1¾" diam.	5	0.6
Eggplant, peeled, diced, cooked	½	cup, ¼ medium (4 oz.)	15	2.5
Green beans, French cut, boiled	½	cup	5	2.0
Green pepper	2	rings	5	0.2
	1	medium—2¾″ × 2½″diam.	15	0.8
Kidney beans, cooked	½	cup	100	9.3
Lentils, dried, uncooked	¼	cup	145	5.6
Lettuce	⅙	head	10	1.4
	6	medium leaves	5	0.7

Food Item	Serving Size	Calories	Dietary Fiber (In Grams)
Mushrooms:			
raw, sliced or chopped	½ cup	5	0.9
canned, drained	½ cup	20	1.8
Okra, raw	½ cup	15	2.6
Onions:			
raw, sliced	½ cup	15	0.7
raw, chopped	1 Tbsp.	0	0.1
boiled	½ cup	15	1.4
spring or green	2 medium	10	0.9
Parsley, fresh, chopped	1 Tbsp.	0	0.3
Peas, green, boiled	½ cup	40	4.2
Peas:			
dried, uncooked	¼ cup	143	8.4
dried, split, uncooked	¼ cup	155	6.0
Pickles:			
dill	1 medium–3¾" × 1¼" diam.	5	1.1
sweet	4 slices	35	0.5
Potatoes:			
baked with skin	1 medium–2½" diam.	130	3.0

boiled, peeled	1 medium	2.7
boiled, sliced	½ cup	1.6
French fried	10 strips	1.6
mashed with milk and butter	½ cup	0.9
Radishes	10 medium	0.5
Sauerkraut, solids and liquid	½ cup	3.3
Spinach, boiled	½ cup	5.7
Sweet potatoes:		
canned, drained	1 cup	4.6
boiled, peeled	1 (5" long × 2" diam.)	3.5
Tomatoes:		
raw	1 medium–2⅗" diam.	2.0
canned, solids and liquid	1 cup	2.2
Tomato juice	½ cup	0
Tomato sauce	½ cup	2.6
Turnips, boiled and mashed	½ cup	3.2
Watercress, fresh, cut	½ cup–5 sprigs	0.6

Food Item	Serving Size		Calories	Dietary Fiber (In Grams)
FRUITS AND FRUIT JUICES				
Apple, unpared	1	small—2½" diam.	50	2.1
	1	medium—3" diam.	75	3.3
Apple juice	½	cup	60	0
Applesauce, canned, unsweetened	½	cup	40	2.6
Apricots	2	medium	20	1.6
Apricots, dried	¼	cup	60	7.8
Banana	½	small—7¾" long	40	1.6
	½	cup slices	60	2.6
Cantaloupe	¼		40	1.6
Cherries, sweet	10	large	30	1.2
	½	cup	35	1.2
Dates, dried	5		90	3.1
Fig	1	medium	30	2.4
Grapefruit	½	whole	20	0.6
Grapefruit, canned, syrup packed	½	cup	75	0.5
Grapefruit juice:				
sweetened	½	cup	65	0
unsweetened	½	cup	50	0
Grapes, seedless	10		20	0.3
	½	cup	50	0.7

Honeydew melon	1	wedge (1/10 melon)	30	1.3
Lemon	1	slice	0	0.5
Lemon juice	1	Tbsp.	5	0
Lemonade, frozen, diluted	1	cup	105	0
Lychees	5		50	0.3
Mango	1		120	3.0
Nectarine	1	medium–2½" diam.	70	3.0
Olives	10	medium	50	2.1
Orange	1	small–2½" diam.	40	2.4
Orange juice	½	cup	55	0
Oranges, mandarin	½	cup	55	0.3
Peach, unpared	1	medium–2½" diam.	35	1.4
	½	cup slices	30	1.2
Peaches, canned halves, light syrup	½	cup	70	1.2
Pear, unpared	1	small–2½" diam.	45	2.6
Pineapple	½	cup	35	0.9
Pineapple:				
canned, heavy syrup	½	cup	100	1.1
canned, in juice	½	cup	50	1.1

Food Item	Serving Size	Calories	Dietary Fiber (In Grams)
Pineapple juice, unsweetened	½ cup	70	0
Plums	2 medium–1″ diam.	10	0.4
Prunes:			
uncooked	2 medium	20	2.0
stewed, unsweetened	½ cup	80	7.8
Raisins	2 Tbsp.	45	1.2
Raspberries	½ cup	15	4.6
Rhubarb, stewed, sweetened	½ cup	55	2.8
Strawberries	½ cup	20	1.7
Tangerine	1 medium–2⅜″ diam.	30	1.6

MEAT, POULTRY, FISH, EGGS

Food Item	Serving Size	Calories	Dietary Fiber (In Grams)
Beef:			
corned	3 ounces	315	0
patty	3 ounces	245	0
rib roast	3 ounces	205	0
roast	3 ounces	175	0
steak	3 ounces	175	0
Chicken:			
dark meat	3 ounces, ⅔ cup chopped	150	0
white meat	3 ounces, ⅔ cup chopped	140	0

Chicken, fried:		
1 drumstick	1.3 ounces	90
1 thigh	2 ounces	120
½ breast	3 ounces	160
Chicken, roasted:		
1 drumstick	1.3 ounces	70
1 thigh	2 ounces	95
½ breast	3 ounces	145
Egg, soft or hard cooked	1 large	80
Fish fillet:		
flounder	3 ounces	120
halibut	3 ounces	110
Fish cakes	3 ounces	160
Fish sticks, breaded	3 ounces	205
Frankfurter	1 (2 ounces)	175
Haddock, breaded	3 ounces	140
Ham:		
lean, baked or roasted	3 ounces	185
boiled, luncheon meat	2 ounces	135
Lamb:		
chop	3 ounces	160
roast	3 ounces	175

Food Item	Serving Size		Calories	Dietary Fiber (In Grams)
Liver:				
beef	3	ounces	150	0
calf	3	ounces	165	0
Meatloaf	3	ounces	170	0
Meat salads:				
chicken	1/3	cup	260	0.3
tuna	1/2	cup	270	0.5
Pork:				
chop	3	ounces	230	0
loin	3	ounces	215	0
sausage	1	ounce	135	0
	1	link	60	0
Salmon:				
steak	3	ounces	155	0
smoked	3	ounces	150	0
Shrimp:				
boiled	3	ounces	100	0
French fried	3	ounces	190	0

NOTE: Meat may be prepared by baking, roasting, broiling or boiling. Serving size refers to the weight of the meat after cooking and after bone, skin and fat have been removed.

Tuna:			
in oil, drained	3	ounces	170	0
in water, drained	3	ounces	110	0
Turkey, roasted:			
dark meat	3	ounces	175	0
white meat	3	ounces	150	0
Veal cutlet	3	ounces	185	0

BREADS

Bread:			
cracked wheat	1	slice	55	2.1
pumpernickel	1	slice	55	1.2
raisin	1	slice	65	0.4
rye	1	slice	60	1.2
white	1	slice	65	0.8
whole wheat	1	slice	50	2.1
Coffeecake	1	piece—2⅝″ × 2¾″ × 1¼″	230	0.7
Frankfurter bun	1	(6″ long, 2″ wide)	120	1.2
Hamburger bun	1	(3½″ diam., 1½″ high)	120	1.2
Pancake, plain or buttermilk	1	(4″ diam., ⅜″ thick)	60	0.5

Food Item	Serving Size		Calories	Dietary Fiber (In Grams)
Roll:				
dinner	1	(3¾" × 2½" × 1¾")	75	0.8
hard, brown	1	(3¾" × 2½" × 1¾")	70	1.5
hard, white	1	(3¾" × 2½" × 1¾")	70	0.8
Taco shell (tortilla)	1		45	0
Rye wafers	3	(3½" long)	65	2.3
Saltines	4		50	0
Waffle, frozen, round	1	squares	120	0.7
CEREALS				
Barley, pearled, uncooked	¼	cup	180	3.3
Kellogg's® All-Bran® cereal	⅓	cup (1 oz.)	70	9.0
Kellogg's® Bran Buds® cereal	⅓	cup (1 oz.)	70	8.0
Kellogg's® Cracklin' Bran® cereal	½	cup (1 oz.)	110	4.0
Kellogg's® 40% Bran Flakes cereal	⅔	cup (1 oz.)	90	4.0
Oatmeal, uncooked	⅓	cup	105	1.9
Rice, white, long grain, cooked	½	cup	125	0.8

PASTA

Egg noodles, boiled	½	cup	110	0
Macaroni or spaghetti, boiled	½	cup	80	0

FATS

Bacon, cooked and drained	2	medium strips	85	0
Butter	1	pat (about 1 tsp.)	35	0
Cream cheese	1	Tbsp.	50	0
Dressings:				
blue cheese, regular	1	Tbsp.	76	0
French style, regular	1	Tbsp.	65	0
French style, low calorie	1	Tbsp.	15	0
Italian style, regular	1	Tbsp.	85	0
Italian style, low calorie	1	Tbsp.	10	0
salad dressing, mayonnaise-type	1	Tbsp.	65	0
thousand island, regular	1	Tbsp.	80	0
Margarine	1	pat (about 1 tsp.)	35	0
Mayonnaise:				
regular	1	Tbsp.	100	0
reduced calorie	1	Tbsp.	40	0
Salad or cooking oil	1	Tbsp.	120	0
Sour cream	1	Tbsp.	25	0

Food Item	Serving Size		Calories	Dietary Fiber (In Grams)
Tartar sauce:				
regular	1	Tbsp.	75	0
low calorie	1	Tbsp.	30	0
White sauce, medium	¼	cup	100	0
SEEDS AND NUTS				
Almonds, shelled	¼	cup	200	5.1
Peanut butter, smooth	2	Tbsp.	200	2.4
Peanuts:				
roasted and salted	¼	cup	205	2.9
Spanish	20		50	0.7
Walnuts:				
chopped pieces	¼	cup	160	1.6
halves	¼	cup	130	1.3
MISCELLANEOUS				
Beer	12	ounces	150	0
Bouillon	1	cup	100	0
	1	cube	5	0
	1	tsp. powder	0	0
Coffee	1	cup	5	0

Corn, popped	1	cup popped	40	0.4
Diet soft drink	12	ounces	0	0
Gelatin dessert, fruit-flavored, prepared				
with water	½	cup	70	0
Honey	1	tsp.	20	0
Jam or preserves	1	tsp.	20	0
Jelly	1	tsp.	20	0
Ketchup	1	Tbsp.	15	0
Maple or cane syrup	1	Tbsp.	50	0
Minestrone, prepared with water	1	cup	55	1.2
Mustard	1	tsp.	5	0
Non-dairy whipped topping	1	Tbsp.	10	0
Pickle relish, sweet	1	Tbsp.	10	0.1
Sugar, white or brown	1	tsp.	15	0
Tea	1	cup	0	0
Vanilla wafers	4	(1⅛″ diam.)	75	0
Vinegar	1	Tbsp.	0	0
Wine:				
dessert	½	cup	165	0
table	½	cup	100	0

Kellogg's® Bran Idea Book™ © 1982 Kellogg Company
Used with permission

INDEX